RETINAL DETACHMENT
DIAGNOSIS
AND
MANAGEMENT

WILLIAM EDMUNDS BENSON, M.D., F.A.C.S.

Associate Surgeon, Wills Eye Hospital
Associate Professor, Department of Ophthalmology, Thomas Jefferson School of Medicine
Senior Surgeon, Children's Hospital of Philadelphia
Attending Surgeon, Chestnut Hill Hospital
Assistant Surgeon, Pennsylvania Hospital
Consultant, Philadelphia Naval Hospital, Philadelphia, Pennsylvania

RETINAL DETACHMENT

DIAGNOSIS AND MANAGEMENT

HARPER & ROW, PUBLISHERS

HAGERSTOWN

Cambridge
New York
Philadelphia
San Francisco

London
Mexico City
São Paulo
Sydney

1817

To "The Penguin"

The authors and publisher have exerted every effort to ensure that drug selection and dosage set forth in this text are in accord with current recommendations and practice at the time of publication. However, in view of ongoing research, changes in government regulations, and the constant flow of information relating to drug therapy and drug reactions, the reader is urged to check the package insert for each drug for any change in indications and dosage and for added warnings and precautions. This is particularly important when the recommended agent is a new and/or infrequently employed drug.

80   81   82   83   84   85   10   9   8   7   6   5   4   3   2   1

RETINAL DETACHMENT: Diagnosis and Management
Copyright © 1980, by Harper & Row, Publishers, Inc.
All rights reserved. No part of this book may be used or reproduced in any manner whatsoever without written permission except in the case of brief quotations embodied in critical articles and reviews. Printed in the United States of America. For information address Medical Department, Harper & Row, Publishers, Inc., 2350 Virginia Avenue, Hagerstown, Maryland 21740

ISBN 0-06-140410-1

Library of Congress Catalog Card Number: 79-20475
Library of Congress Cataloging in Publication Data
Benson, William Edmunds.
  Retinal detachment.

  Bibliography
  Includes index.
  1. Retinal detachment.   2. Retina—Surgery.
RE603.B46   617.7'3   79-20475
ISBN 0-06-140410-1

CONTENTS

Contents

FOREWORD

Sixty years ago, Gonin published the first rational approach to the treatment of rhegmatogenous retinal detachment: closure of the retinal breaks. Thirty years ago, Custodis supplemented Gonin's principles with the introduction of scleral-choroidal indentation at the site of the retinal breaks.

In the United States, the widespread use of the Schepens binocular indirect ophthalmoscope and the Goldmann three-mirror lens has greatly enhanced the preoperative and postoperative evaluation of eyes with the retina detached. Today, few, if any, retinal detachments are considered inoperable and the success rate in several large reported series exceeds 90%.

With the introduction of vitreous surgery by Kasner and Machemer, a new approach has been added to the retinal surgeon's armamentarium.

It seems appropriate that the time has come for some of us to take a breath and try to condense man's accomplishments to date so that the upcoming generation of ophthalmologists can easily learn the present "state of the art" and the important milestones in these achievements.

Dr. Benson is eminently qualified to undertake this mission since his educational program has exposed him to several different retinal programs, and his personal experience has been more than sufficient to allow him to sort out for himself the present "state of the art".

This book, *Retinal Detachment, Diagnosis and Management,* is well organized, concisely written, and appropriately illustrated, representing an accurate account of retinal surgery as seen in the perspective of 1979. Certain problems, such as indications for prophylactic treatment, and the incidence of retinal detachment when the zonular-lens capsule diaphragm has been left intact during cataract surgery, remain to be studied and resolved in the future.

Edward W. D. Norton, M.D.

PREFACE

This book is intended to provide residents, fellows, and practitioners of ophthalmology with a guide to the diagnosis and management of retinal detachment. Basic principles are stressed to give the reader the knowledge necessary to cope with individual cases not specifically discussed. The first three chapters discuss the basic mechanism and pathophysiology of primary rhegmatogenous retinal detachment and the conditions that predispose to it. A historical survey of theories and treatments is presented in Chapter Four. Chapters Five through Nine deal with fundus examination, differential diagnosis, and surgical management. Chapter Ten provides guidelines for prophylactic treatment of retinal breaks.

The techniques outlined reflect my training at Washington University in St. Louis and at the Bascom Palmer Eye Institute in Miami. However, to the best of my ability, I have tried to present impartially both sides of controversial issues.

I am indebted to many individuals who have helped to make this publication possible. First, I would like to thank my teachers: Dr. Harold Spalter at Columbia University, who fostered my interest in ophthalmology; Drs. Edward Okun, Glen Johnston, Isaac Boniuk, and Neva Arribas at Washington University; and Drs. Edward Norton, Victor Curtin, Donald Gass, Robert Machemer, Guy O'Grady, Mary Lou Louis, Donald Nicholson, and George Blankenship at the Bascom Palmer Eye Institute. I am indebted to the ophthalmologists of the Delaware Valley and to those on the staffs of the Wills Eye Hospital and the Scheie Eye Institute for referring the patients whose photographs appear. The fundus photographs were taken by Ms. Laurel Weeney and Messrs. Donald Morozin, William Nyberg, and Terry Tomer. Mr. David Silva and Ms. Jo Hoffman took the operating room photographs and, with Ms. Angeles Roca, prepared the illustrations. Most of the artwork was drawn by Ms. Laurel Cook. Ms. Fleur Weinberg and Ms. Gloria Lewis verified the references. The manuscript was patiently typed and retyped by Mss. Mary Kennedy, Edie Rosen, Lucy Freedman, Barbara Armstrong, and Thea Fischer. Photocopying was done by Mss. Joy Beetem, Susan Erickson, Amy Nearing, and Mary Jo Young. I am grateful to Drs. Robert Machemer, Horst Laqua, Myron Yanoff, Ben Fine, John Clarkson, W. Richard Green, Darcy Massof, Edward W. D. Norton, Gerry Shields, Sheldon Kaplan, Charles Schepens, Lov Sarin, William Annesley, and George Blankenship for lending me slides and prints. Drs. M. Gilbert Grand, Dwain Fuller, Louis Lobes, and Alan Crandall reviewed the manuscript and made many useful suggestions. Steve Felton, Paul Pender, Elizabeth Miller, Andrew Levin and Greg Genzheimer helped with the proofreading. Special thanks go to Dr. William Tasman for his invaluable ideas, illustrations, and moral support. Finally, I would like to thank my wife, Linda, who spent countless hours editing and rewriting the text. Any stylistic merit this book may have should be credited to her.

William Edmunds Benson, M.D.

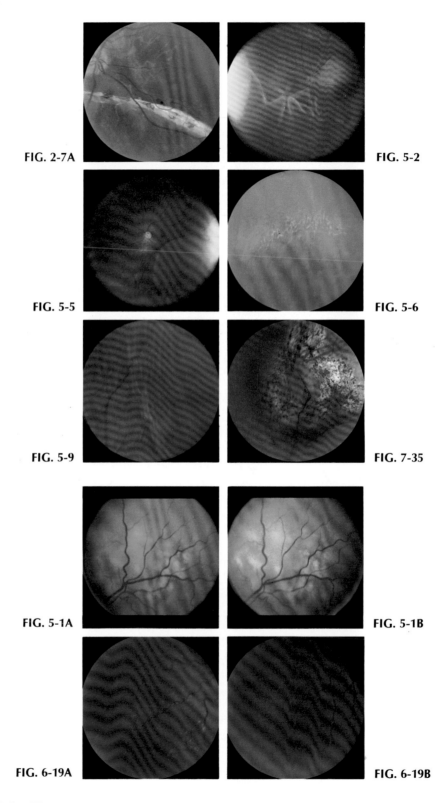

FIG. 2-7A

FIG. 5-2

FIG. 5-5

FIG. 5-6

FIG. 5-9

FIG. 7-35

FIG. 5-1A

FIG. 5-1B

FIG. 6-19A

FIG. 6-19B

COLOR PLATE 1

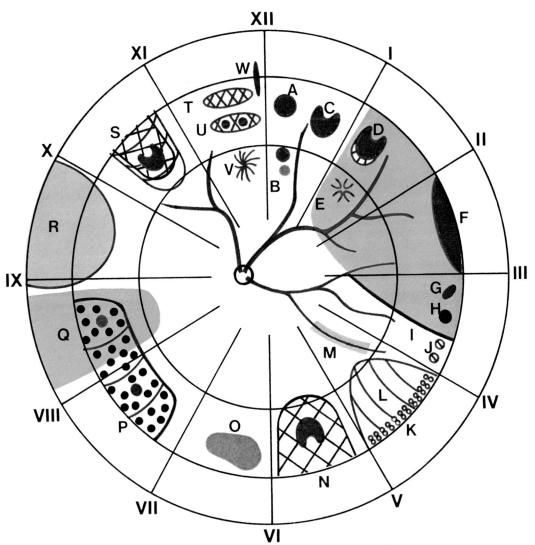

FIG. 6-16. Schematic drawing of retinal findings. Arteries and intraretinal or subretinal hemorrhages are red. Veins are blue. Red outlined by blue indicates retinal breaks. Attached retina is white. Detached retina is blue. Intraretinal and subretinal exudates are yellow. Chorioretinal scarring (pigment epithelial proliferation) is black. Any choroidal mass or indentation is brown. (Clearly, a label is required to distinguish a choroidal detachment from a malignant melanoma.) Anything in the vitreous (hemorrhage, foreign body, etc.) is green. Here, too, a label is often required. (A) round hole; (B) operculated tear; (C) flap tear; (D) flap tear with posteriorly rolled edge; (E) fixed fold; (F) retinal dialysis (disinsertion); (G) retinal hemorrhage; (H) intraretinal pigmentation; (I) demarcation line; (J) cobblestones; (K) peripheral cystoid degeneration; (L) senile retinoschisis; (M) exudate along a retinal artery; (N) flap tear surrounded by cryotherapy scarring; (O) vitreous opacity (needs label); (P) two round holes on a circumferential scleral buckle surrounded by diathermy scars. Superiorly, the retina has redetached; (Q) detachment of non-pigmented epithelium of the pars plana; (R) choroidal mass (needs label); (S) flap surrounded by cryotherapy scarring on a radical scleral buckle; (T) lattice degeneration; (U) lattice degeneration with atrophic round holes; (V) votex vein ampulla; (W) meridional fold.

COLOR PLATE 2

1

PRIMARY
RETINAL
DETACHMENT

A retinal detachment is an accumulation of fluid in the potential space between the sensory retina and the retinal pigment epithelium. In a rhegmatogenous (Greek *rhegma*, rent) retinal detachment, the fluid gains access to this space through a break in the retina. A primary, or spontaneous, retinal detachment is a rhegmatogenous detachment in which the retinal break has not been caused by an antecedent event (such as trauma) or condition (such as proliferative retinopathy). Primary detachments are usually preceded by posterior vitreous detachment.

POSTERIOR VITREOUS DETACHMENT

MECHANISM

A meshwork of collagen fibers occupies the vitreous cavity. Hyaluronic acid molecules are interspersed between the fibers, supporting them. The fibers are firmly attached to the retina and to the epithelium of the pars plana for a few millimeters to each side of the ora serrata. This area is called the vitreous base (Fig. 1-1). Less firm adhesions are found at the optic disc, at the macula, along retinal blood vessels,[27] and around areas of chorioretinal scarring. A yet weaker adhesion exists between the vitreous and the internal limiting membrane of the retina.

As one gets older, the hyaluronic acid concentration decreases, depriving the collagen fibers of their support and causing them to aggregate. In some cases, the collagen meshwork collapses and moves forward, separating the posterior vitreous from the internal limiting membrane of the retina. This phenomenon, called posterior vitreous detachment (PVD), was found in autopsy studies in approximately 80 per cent of aphakic eyes and in 31 per cent of phakic eyes of individuals over 65 years of age.[15] The incidence is higher in individuals with aphakic eyes because the removal of the lens permits the hyaluronic acid to pass more easily into the anterior chamber and thence out of the eye.[23] Clinical studies[13, 17] report a higher incidence of posterior vitreous detachment than do the autopsy studies. The difficulty of clinically ascertaining whether or not a thin layer of vitreous is adherent to the posterior retina probably accounts for the erroneous figures of the clinical studies.

SYMPTOMS

As the vitreous collapses, it can tear away epipapillary glial tissue, which is perceived by the patient as a "floater," often described as a cobweb or a fly

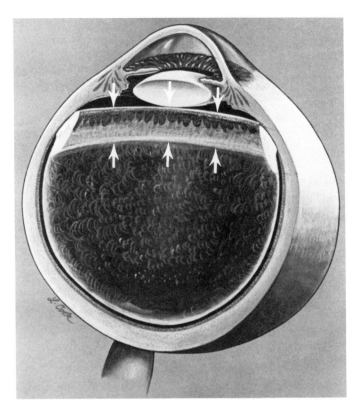

FIG. 1-1. Vitreous base (*between arrows*) straddling the ora serrata.

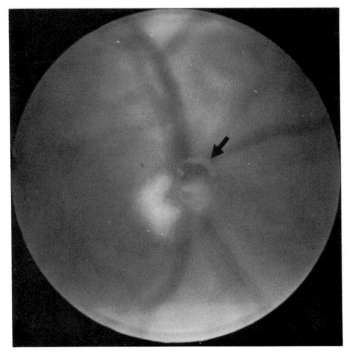

FIG. 1-2. Epipapillary glial tissue (*arrow*) torn free by the collapsing vitreous.

(Fig. 1-2). Vitreous traction on the peripheral retina can cause photopsia, the subjective impression of flashing lights ("flashes"), which is seen by about one-third of the patients who present with acute posterior vitreous detachment.[17, 19, 22, 35] Patients are more aware of the light flashes in dim illumination. They may also see flashing colored lights. Interestingly, more females than males report photopsia. In addition to the typical central floater, the patient may notice a "shower of floaters," "reddish smoke," or simply blurred vision. These are all symptoms of vitreous hemorrhage, which is found in 13 to 19 per cent of patients with acute PVD.[17, 19, 34, 35] The hemorrhage results when papillary or retinal vessels are torn by vitreous traction or when retinal vessels crossing retinal tears are avulsed.

CLINICAL FINDINGS

From 8 to 15 per cent of all patients presenting with acute symptomatic posterior vitreous detachment have a retinal tear.[17, 19, 34, 35] As many as one-half of these patients have more than one tear.[21] Most of the tears are located superiorly. Although light flashes are felt to be a sign of retinal traction, patients with flashes do not have a higher incidence of retinal tears than do patients without flashes.[19]

Vitreous hemorrhage is an ominous sign. Acute PVD with vitreous hemorrhage has a 70 per cent incidence of retinal tears, as opposed to a 2 to 4 per cent incidence in acute PVD without hemorrhage.[17, 19, 34, 35]

Pigmented cells ("tobacco dust") in the vitreous of patients with no previous ocular surgery are practically pathognomic of retinal detachment or retinal tear.[12, 26, 33]

Almost all patients with retinal detachment have posterior vitreous detachment, but 50 per cent of retinal detachment patients never experience flashes or floaters, presenting instead with the symptoms of detachment: visual field loss or decreased visual acuity.[8, 22]

MANAGEMENT

All patients with symptoms of PVD should be examined with indirect ophthalmoscopy and scleral depression. The examiner, utilizing the Hruby or Goldmann lens, should carefully inspect the vitreous for hemorrhage. If there is no hemorrhage and the symptoms have been present for 3 or more months, the patient should be reexamined in 3 months. If, however, the patient has vitreous hemorrhage or acute symptomatic PVD of recent onset, he should be reexamined in 1 or 2 weeks and then at regular intervals for 6 months, after which development of a retinal detachment is unlikely.[34]

All patients should be instructed to return immediately if they notice an increase in floaters; this might indicate increased vitreous traction and a possible retinal tear. Patients with PVD should also be taught the symptoms of retinal detachment and told to report immediately if they perceive a "curtain" or "shadow" in the peripheral field of vision.

Patients with a gross vitreous hemorrhage should be reexamined at one or two week intervals until the entire periphery can be observed. Ultrasonography is an invaluable diagnostic tool for evaluation of patients with vitreous hemorrhage when fundus examination is impossible. Patients with a dense vitreous hemorrhage of unknown etiology through which fundus details cannot be seen should be hospitalized for bedrest and bilateral patching for 2 or 3 days. The head of the bed should be elevated. In most cases, the hemorrhage will clear sufficiently to permit retinal examination.

Patients with peripheral punctate intraretinal hemorrhages should be followed very carefully.[18, 35] Such hemorrhages indicate vitreous traction and may mark the site of a later tear.

RETINAL BREAKS

Throughout this book, the following terminology will be used: a retinal *break* is any full-thickness retinal defect; a *tear* is a break caused by vitreous traction; a *hole* is an atrophic round break.

TEARS

When the vitreous body collapses, it usually separates easily from the retina except at the vitreous base. If there are no posterior vitreoretinal adhesions, a retinal tear is unlikely. On the other hand, if there is strong focal vitreous traction (Fig. 1-3), a retinal tear can result (Fig. 1-4). Strong posterior vitreous adhesions may exist perivascularly,[27] at posterior extensions of the vitreous base,[10] or at vitreoretinal tufts,[10] pigmented spots,[6] meridional folds,[29] enclosed ora bays,[28] or lattice degeneration (Fig. 1-5).[32, 39]

As the vitreous collapses, traction on these adhesions may pull a strip of retina anteriorly, causing a *flap* (horseshoe) tear (Fig. 1-6). The posterior edge of the tear is its *apex*. The area where the torn strip (*flap*) remains adherent to the retina is its *base*. The *horns* are the anterior extensions of the tear. If a piece of the retina is torn completely free from the retinal surface, it is called an *operculum*, and the tear is said to be *operculated* (Fig. 1-7).

ROUND HOLES

Focal retinal atrophy can result in a full-thickness retinal break (Fig. 1-8). Atrophic round holes are frequently found in areas of lattice degeneration (Fig. 1-9). Round holes are less likely to cause retinal detachment than are tears with associated vitreous traction (see chapter 10, Prophylactic Therapy).

SENILE RETINOSCHISIS

Atrophic holes may develop in both walls of senile retinoschisis cavities. Outer wall holes can give rise to retinal detachment even if the inner wall is intact (see chapter 5, Differential Diagnosis).

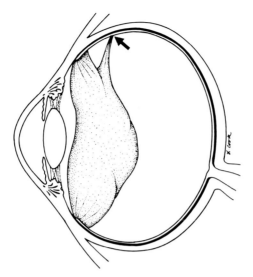

FIG. 1-3. Posterior vitreous detachment with vitreoretinal adhesion (*arrow*) posterior to the vitreous base. The strong focal traction may cause a retinal tear.

FIG. 1-4. Flap (horseshoe) tear of the retina. Note vitreous (V) adherent to the flap. PAS × 40. (From Yanoff M, Fine BS: *Ocular Pathology. A Text and Atlas.* Hagerstown, Harper and Row, 1975.)

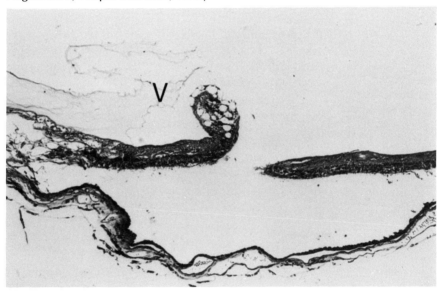

DIALYSIS (DISINSERTION)

A retinal dialysis (Greek *dia*, apart; *lysis*, dissolution) is a separation of the sensory retina from the non-pigmented epithelium of the pars plana at the ora serrata (Fig. 1-10). Dialyses may be spontaneous or may result from blunt trauma (see chapter 3, Predisposing Conditions). They are most commonly located in the inferotemporal quadrant. A tendency toward dialysis may be

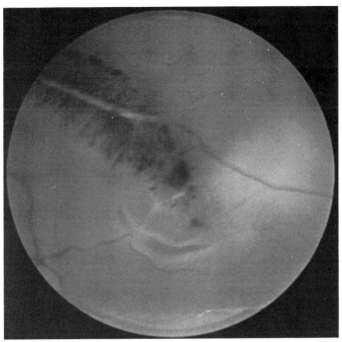

FIG. 1-5. Crescentic tear caused by vitreous traction at the end of an area of pigmented lattice degeneration. The retina is detached.

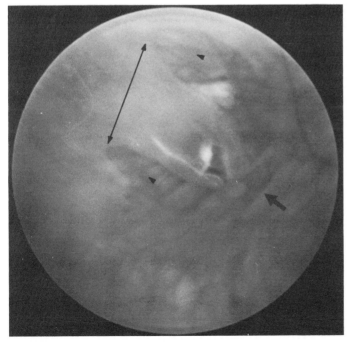

FIG. 1-6. Flap (horseshoe) tear caused by vitreous traction on the posterior edge of a small area of lattice degeneration. Arrow indicates the apex; solid line, the base; and arrowheads, the horns.

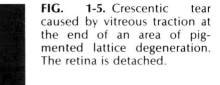

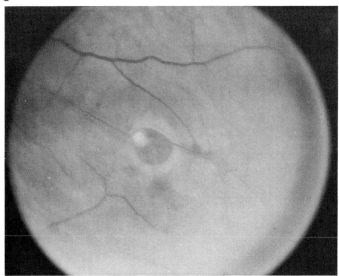

FIG. 1-7. Operculated retinal tear. Notice that the retinal artery is attached to the operculum. (Courtesy George W. Blankenship, M.D.)

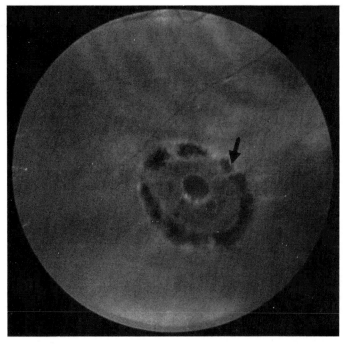

FIG. 1-8. Atrophic round hole surrounded by a small rim of subretinal fluid and a pigmented demarcation line (*arrow*).

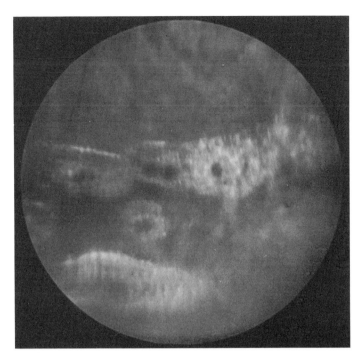

FIG. 1-9. Multiple rows of lattice degeneration with atrophic round holes.

FIG. 1-10. A retinal dialysis. The sensory retina (R) is separated from the non-pigmented epithelium of the pars plana at the ora serrata (*arrows*). (Courtesy W. Richard Green, M.D.)

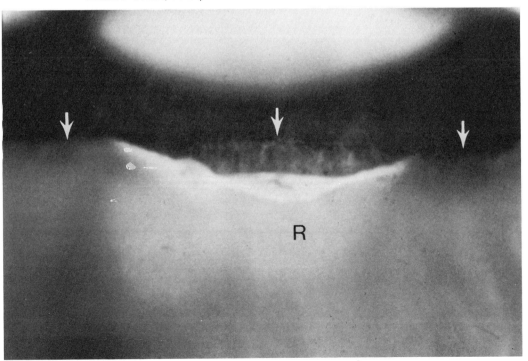

hereditary.[37] Technically, dialyses are not retinal breaks, but they do expose the subretinal space to liquid vitreous and may thereby cause a retinal detachment.

WHAT KEEPS THE RETINA ATTACHED?

Retinal detachment results when liquid vitreous passes through a retinal break to the potential space between the sensory retina and the pigment epithelium. The vast majority of persons with retinal breaks, however, never develop a retinal detachment. The mechanism by which the retina remains attached, even in the presence of a break, is not known. Three current credible theories are discussed below.

ACID MUCOPOLYSACCHARIDE

The acid mucopolysaccharide (AMPS) found between the sensory retina and the pigment epithelium[40] may act as a "biological glue," binding these surfaces together.[7,41] It is also possible that this viscous polymer prevents the liquid vitreous from gaining access to the potential subretinal space.

RETINAL PIGMENT EPITHELIAL CELL SHEATHS

In rabbits, the force required to mechanically peel the retina from the pigment epithelium is markedly decreased immediately after death,[41] indicating that active forces play a role in keeping the retina attached. There is good evidence that pigment epithelial cells actually hold the retina in place mechanically. Experimentally induced detachments have demonstrated a strong adhesion between photoreceptor outer segments and their pigment epithelial sheaths. Mechanical peeling of the retina from the pigment epithelium in vivo stretches and deforms the sheaths, whereas peeling in vitro does not.[41] Electron microscopy shows that the sheaths surround and are closely apposed to the outer segments.[16,30] Moreover, they exert a contractile force which phagocytizes the outer segments.[30] Actin has recently been identified in these sheaths.[5]

HYDROSTATIC PRESSURE

In non-drainage procedures, once the retinal break is closed, the subretinal fluid is promptly absorbed. It is not known whether the subretinal fluid is actively pumped out by the pigment epithelium or whether it is drawn through the pigment epithelium by the osmotic pressure of the protein-rich choroid.[2] Removal of the fluid lowers the hydrostatic pressure in the subretinal space relative to that in the vitreous. The vitreous pressure then flattens the retina. The same mechanism may help to keep the retina attached.[2,9]

INCIDENCE OF RETINAL DETACHMENT

Phakic, non-traumatic retinal detachment occurs in approximately five to ten persons per 100,000 population per year.[3,14,24,31] The inclusion of traumatic retinal detachment only slightly increases this figure. Partly because males are more likely to suffer trauma than females, they have a higher incidence of retinal detachment (61 per cent versus 39 per cent).[1] For unknown reasons, Blacks have a lower incidence of retinal detachment than do Caucasians.[4,38]

Early reports from large referral centers indicated that the incidence of bilateral retinal detachment was 20 to 25 per cent.[11,23a,25] Because of the referral nature of these institutions, this figure was much higher for their patient population than for the general population. Many of the patients were referred for treatment of the second eye. More recent studies have avoided this error; they report the incidence of bilateral retinal detachment to be about 10 per cent.[6,8,20,36]

REFERENCES

1. **Ashrafzadeh MT, Schepens CL, Elzeneiny IT, Moura R, Morse P, Kraushar MF:** Aphakic and phakic retinal detachment. Arch Ophthalmol 89:476, 1973
2. **Bill A:** Blood circulation and fluid dynamics in the eye. Physiol Rev 55:383, 1975
3. **Bohringer HR:** Statistisches zur Haufigkeit und Risiko der Netzhautablösung. Ophthalmologica 131:331, 1956
4. **Brown PR, Thomas RD:** The incidence of primary retinal detachment in the Negro. Am J Ophthalmol 60:109, 1965
5. **Burnside B, Laties A:** Actin filaments in apical projections of the primate pigmented epithelial cell. Invest Ophthalmol 15:570, 1976
6. **Davis MD:** Natural history of retinal breaks. Arch Ophthalmol 92:183, 1974
7. **deGuillebon H, Zauberman H:** Experimental retinal detachment. Biophysical aspects of retinal peeling and stretching. Arch Ophthalmol 87:545, 1972
8. **Delaney WV Jr, Oates RP:** Retinal detachment in the second eye. Arch Ophthalmol 96:629, 1978
9. **Fatt I, Shantinath K:** Flow conductivity of retina and its role in retinal adhesion. Exp Eye Res 12:218, 1971
10. **Foos RY:** Vitreous base, retinal tufts, and retinal tears: pathogenic relationships. In Pruett RC, Regan CDJ (eds): Retina Congress. New York, Appleton-Century-Crofts, 1972, 259–280
11. **Funder W:** Das Schicksel der einseitig an Netzhautablösung Erblinden. Klin Monatsbl Angenheilkd 129:330, 1956
12. **Hamilton AM, Taylor W:** Significance of pigment granules in the vitreous. Br J Ophthalmol 56:700, 1972
13. **Hauer Y, Barkay S:** Vitreous detachment in aphakic eyes. Br J Ophthalmol 48:341, 1964
14. **Haut J, Massin M:** Fréquence des décollements de retine dans la population française. Pourcentage des décollements bilateraux. Arch Ophthalmologie 35:533, 1975
15. **Heller MD, Straatsma BR, Foos RY:** Detachment of the posterior vitreous in phakic and aphakic eyes. Mod Probl Ophthalmol 10:23, 1972
16. **Hogan MJ, Alvarado JA, Weddell JE:** Histology of the Human Eye. Philadelphia, WB Saunders, 1971, pp 405–421
17. **Jaffe NS:** Vitreous detachments. In The Vitreous in Clinical Ophthalmology. St. Louis, CV Mosby, 1969, pp 83–98
18. **Kanski JJ:** Complications of acute posterior vitreous detachment. Am J Ophthalmol 80:44, 1975
19. **Lindner B:** Acute posterior vitreous detachment and its retinal complications. Acta Ophthalmol [Suppl] 87:1, 1977
20. **Merin S, Feiler V, Hyams M, Ivry M, Krakowski D, Landau L, Maythar B, Michaelson IC, Scharf J, Schul A, Ser I:** The fate of the fellow eye in retinal detachment. Am J Ophthalmol 71:477, 1971

21. **Morse PH, Scheie HG:** Prophylactic cryotherapy of retinal breaks. Arch Ophthalmol 92:204, 1974

22 **Morse PH, Scheie HG, Aminlari A:** Light flashes as a clue to retinal disease. Arch Ophthalmol 91:179, 1974

23. **Österlin S:** Vitreous changes after cataract extraction. In Freeman HM, Hirose T, Schepens CL (eds): Vitreous Surgery and Advances in Fundus Diagnosis and Treatment. New York, Appleton-Century-Crofts, 1977, pp 15–21

24. **Paufique L:** The present status of the treatment of retinal detachment. Trans Ophthalmol Soc UK 69:221, 1959

25. **Rintelen F:** Zur Frange der Hänfigkeit der Netzhautablösung and zum Phänomen kompensatorisch—gerontologischer Progresse. Ophthalmologica 143:291, 1962

26. **Shafer DM:** Comment. In Schepens CL, Regan CDJ (eds): Controversial Aspects of the Management of Retinal Detachment. Boston, Little, Brown, 1965, p 51

27. **Spencer LM, Foos RY:** Paravascular vitreoretinal attachments. Role in retinal tears. Arch Ophthalmol 84:557, 1970

28. **Spencer LM, Foos RY, Straatsma BR:** Enclosed bays of the ora serrata. Arch Ophthalmol 83:421, 1970

29. **Spencer LM, Foos RY, Straatsma BR:** Meridional folds, meridional complexes and associated abnormalities of the peripheral retina. Am J Ophthalmol 70:697, 1970

30. **Spitznas M, Hogan MJ:** Outer segments of photoreceptors and the retinal pigment epithelium. Inter-relationship in the human eye. Arch Ophthalmol 84:810, 1970

31. **Stein R, Feller-Ofry V, Romano A:** The effect of treatment in the prevention of retinal detachment. In Michaelson IC, Berman ER (eds): Causes and Prevention of Blindness. New York, Academic Press, 1972, pp 409–410

32. **Straatsma BR, Zeegen PD, Foos RY, Feman SS, Shabo AL:** Lattice degeneration of the retina. Am J Ophthalmol 77:619, 1974

33. **Stratford T:** Comment. In Schepens CL, Regan CDJ (eds): Controversial Aspects of the Management of Retinal Detachment. Boston, Little, Brown, 1965, p 51

34. **Tabotabo MD, Benson WE:** Posterior vitreous detachment. (in press)

35. **Tasman WS:** Posterior vitreous detachment and peripheral retinal breaks. Trans Am Acad Ophthalmol Otolaryngol 72:217, 1968

36. **Törnquist R:** Bilateral retinal detachment. Acta Ophthalmol 41:126, 1963

37. **Verdaguer TJ, Rojas B, Lechuga M:** Genetical studies in non-traumatic retinal dialyses. Mod Probl Ophthalmol 15:34, 1975

38. **Weiss H, Tasman WS:** Rhegmatogenous retinal detachments in blacks. Ann Ophthalmol 10:799, 1978

39. **Yanoff M, Fine BS:** Ocular Pathology. Hagerstown, Harper & Row, 1975, pp 455–462

40. **Zimmerman LE, Eastham AB:** Acid mucopolysaccharide in the retinal pigment epithelial and visual cell layer of the developing mouse eye. Am J Ophthalmol 47:488, 1959

41. **Zauberman H, deGuillebon H:** Retinal traction in vivo and postmortem. Arch Ophthalmol 87:549, 1972

2

PATHOPHYSIOLOGY

EARLY RETINAL DETACHMENT

Since very few human eyes with early retinal detachment have been studied histologically, our knowledge is largely derived from experimental retinal detachment in other primates.[25] In the first few days after the retina has been experimentally detached, protein synthesis is decreased[22] and intraretinal edema, most pronounced in the inner nuclear layer, appears (Fig. 2-1).[19, 25] The edema later causes folding of the outer retina. On ophthalmoscopy, the edema and folding are manifested by decreased retinal transparency and irregular corrugations (Fig. 2-2).[19, 25]

The earliest change seen in the photoreceptors is a loss of the horizontal orientation of the discs in the outer segments.[10, 11] Later, the amount of disc material decreases.[10, 11] Since the retinal circulation remains intact, and since the degree of retinal degeneration is proportional to the height of the detachment, it is felt that the above changes are caused by separation of the retina from the pigment epithelium and/or choroid.[19]

Initially, the retinal pigment epithelial cells under the detached retina become larger and proliferate.[8, 10, 19] Some cells separate from Bruch's membrane and float in the subretinal fluid.[19] Clumps of pigment epithelial cells proliferating on the outer surface of the retina are seen clinically as subretinal white dots (Fig. 2-3).[15, 19, 25]

As soon as the detachment is total, the electroretinogram is unrecordable.[6, 17] The electrooculogram is markedly reduced.[17]

LONGSTANDING RETINAL DETACHMENT

The longer the retina remains detached, the more it atrophies. There is necrosis and drop out of cells in all retinal layers (Fig. 2-4). If massive periretinal proliferation does not develop, the retina becomes semitransparent and smooth (Fig. 2-5). Occasionally, large intraretinal cystoid spaces may be seen histologically (Fig. 2-6).[19, 37] The pigment epithelium undergoes atrophy and depigmentation.[8] In retinal detachments of at least 3 months' duration, retinal pigment epithelial cells can proliferate and undergo metaplasia at the junction of attached and detached retina,[8] forming what is clinically known as a demarcation line. The metaplastic cells may produce a fibrous adhesion between the retina and the pigment epithelium; in 23 per cent of cases with demarcation lines, the adhesion is strong enough to prevent progression of the detachment (Fig. 2-7A). In the other 77 per cent, the detachment advances through the demarcation line (Fig. 2-7B).

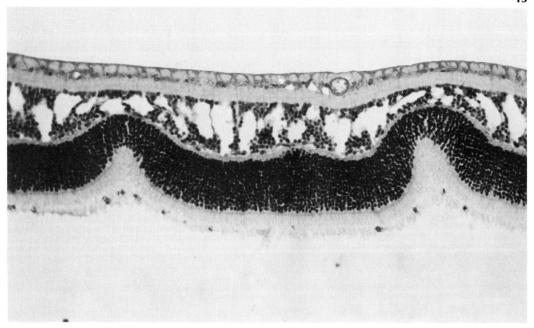

FIG. 2-1. Detachment of 1 week's duration. Edema causes folding of the outer retina. The clinical result is the corrugated appearance seen in Fig. 2-2 (PAS × 190). (Machemer R: Experimental retinal detachment in the owl monkey: II. Histology of retina and pigment epithelium. Am J Ophthalmol 66:396, 1968. Copyright 1968, Ophthalmic Publishing Co)

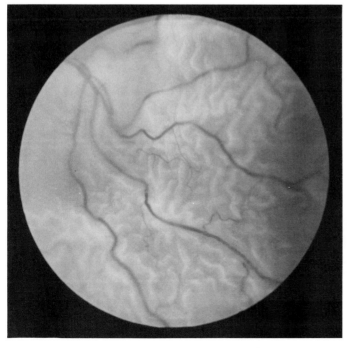

FIG. 2-2. Rhegmatogenous retinal detachment. Corrugated appearance is caused by intraretinal edema.

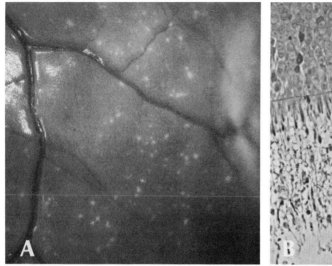
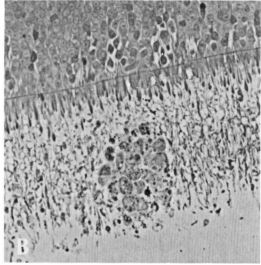

FIG. 2-3. Four-week-old detachment. Left, white retroretinal dots visible through the retina (× 25). Right, dots consist of clusters of pigment epithelial macrophages (phase contrast, × 250). (Laqua H, Machemer R: Clinical-pathological correlation in massive periretinal proliferation. Am J Ophthalmol 80:913, 1975. Copyright 1975, Ophthalmic Publishing Co)

FIG. 2-4. Chronic retinal detachment shows marked degeneration and thinning of outer retinal layers. (Yanoff M, Fine BS: *Ocular Pathology. A Text and Atlas.* Hagerstown, Harper & Row, 1975)

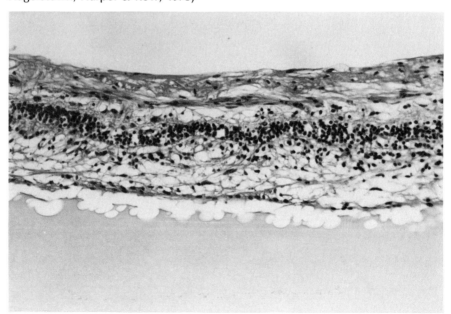

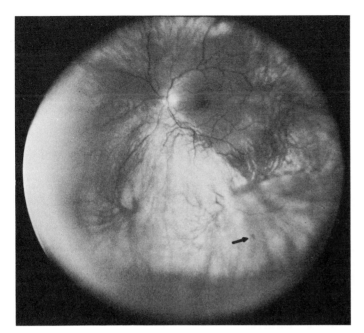

FIG. 2-5. Longstanding inferotemporal retinal detachment without massive periretinal proliferation. The thin retina is semitransparent and smooth. The arrow indicates a round hole. There is a thin demarcation line at the superior edge of the detachment.

FIG. 2-6. Fourteen-week-old detachment. Large cystoid spaces and loss of cells in inner and outer nuclear layer (PAS, × 190). (Machemer, R: Experimental retinal detachment in the owl monkey: II. Histology of the retina and pigment epithelium. Am J Ophthalmol 66:396, 1968. Copyright 1968, Ophthalmic Publishing Co)

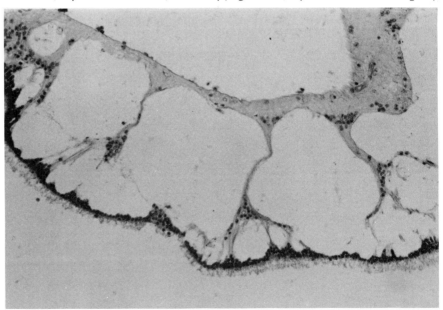

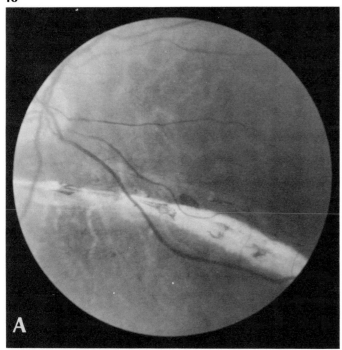

FIG. 2-7. (*A*) Thick demarcation line. It appears white because the metaplastic pigment epithelial cells have become depigmented and have also produced basement membrane material. Notice also the atrophic pigment epithelium inferior to the demarcation line.

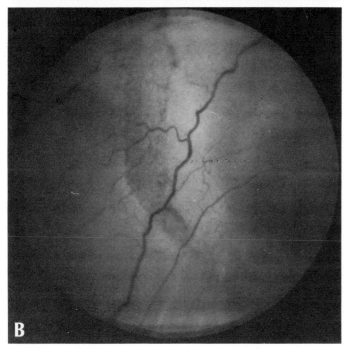

(*B*) Pigmented demarcation line in detached retina. Retina inside (on right of) demarcation line is thinner and smoother than the more recently detached retina outside the demarcation line.

SUBRETINAL FLUID

In rhegmatogenous retinal detachment of recent onset, the protein content of the subretinal fluid is considerably lower than that of plasma.[34] In addition, the subretinal fluid contians hyaluronic acid,[5] which is a component of the vitreous but not of plasma. These facts support the theory that in early retinal detachment liquid vitreous passes through the retinal break, elevating the retina. With increasing duration of the retinal detachment, the composition of the subretinal fluid becomes more and more like that of plasma. The total protein content increases, as does the concentration of enzymes which are normally found only in plasma.[9] There are two possible routes by which plasma components may enter the subretinal fluid. They may pass through the retinal blood vessels, which become more permeable in retinal detachment,[31] or through the pigment epithelium, which degenerates under the detached retina.

The viscosity of the subretinal fluid increases as the protein accumulates. Fluid drained from a detachment of recent onset is very watery, whereas the fluid found in longstanding retinal detachments is quite viscous. Even when all the retinal holes are completely sealed, it may take months for this viscous fluid to be absorbed. It is not known whether the delayed absorption of fluid is caused by its increased viscosity and osmolarity or by degeneration of the pigment epithelium and/or choriocapillaris.

RETINAL RECOVERY AFTER REATTACHMENT

Unless the retina has undergone severe atrophy, recovery after reattachment is remarkably rapid. Within hours of reattachment, protein synthesis is increased and regeneration of the outer segments begins.[13, 22, 23] The electroretinogram may be recordable within 5 hours.[6] Rod outer segments recover faster than do cone outer segments.[12] Intraretinal edema begins to decrease within hours and is nearly completely resolved within 9 days (Fig. 2-8). The electroretinogram continues to improve for 12 weeks,[6] by which time the outer segments are histologically normal.[12, 20] In humans, visual acuity may continue to improve for a year or longer.

MASSIVE PERIRETINAL PROLIFERATION

In many retinal detachments, glial and/or pigment epithelial cells proliferate on either or both surfaces of the retina and/or on vitreous strands, a process known as periretinal proliferation (PP). In extreme cases, the proliferating cells form extensive membranes which can contract, pulling the retina into multiple fixed folds and preventing reattachment (Fig. 2-9). Machemer[21, 24] proposed the term "massive periretinal proliferation" (MPP) to replace the terms "massive vitreous retraction" (MVR) and "massive preretinal retraction" (MPR), both of which fail to completely describe the ubiquitous proliferations.

The cells composing the vitreal membranes are metaplastic retinal pigment epithelial cells which are capable of producing collagen.[2, 3, 24, 26, 27, 30] Transvitreal

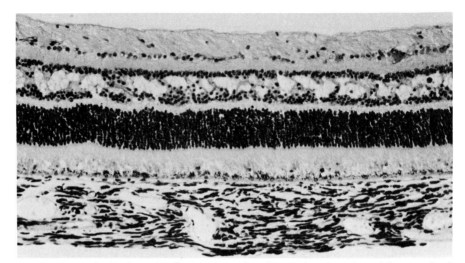

FIG. 2-8. Residual edema in the inner nuclear layer of a nine-day-old reattached retina. (PAS, × 590) (Machemer R: Experimental retinal detachment in the owl monkey. 4. The reattached retina. Am J Ophthalmol 66:1075, 1968. Copyright 1968, Ophthalmic Publishing Co)

FIG. 2-9. Eye with clinical diagnosis of massive periretinal proliferation following unsuccessful retinal detachment surgery. (*A*) The transvitreal portion of the membrane (arrowhead) holds the retina in a funnel shape. The preretinal portion (*arrows*) causes fixed folds (hematoxylin and eosin, × 10). (*B*) Higher power showing thick fibrous preretinal membrane (between arrows) (hemotoxylin and eosin, × 320). (Clarkson JG, Green WR, Massof D: A histopathologic review of 168 cases of preretinal membrane. Am J Ophthalmol 84:1, 1977. Copyright 1977, Ophthalmic Publishing Co)

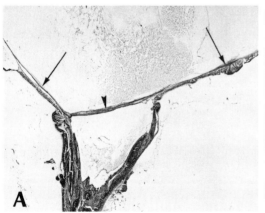 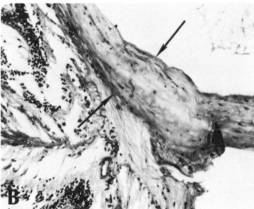

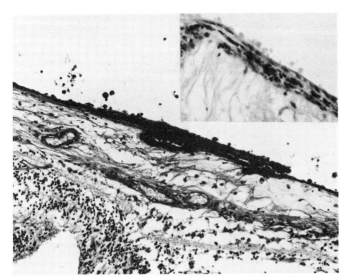

FIG. 2-10. Densely pigmented preretinal membrane is composed of retinal pigment epithelial cells (hematoxylin and eosin, × 160). Inset illustrates the laminated appearance of the membrane with alternate areas of pigment epithelium and basement membrane (partially bleached, hematoxylin and eosin, × 350). (Clarkson JG, Green WR, Massof D: A histopathologic review of 168 cases of preretinal membrane. Am J Ophthalmol 84:1, 1977. Copyright 1977, Ophthalmic Publishing Co)

FIG. 2-11. Small preretinal glial membrane connected to the retina by a thin bridge of tissue. (Arrowheads mark the internal limiting membrane of the retina.) A retinal cell is migrating out of the retina (*arrow*) (PAS, × 400). (Laqua H, Machemer R: Glial cell proliferation in retinal detachment [massive periretinal proliferation]. Am J Ophthalmol 80:602, 1975. Copyright 1975, Ophthalmic Publishing Co)

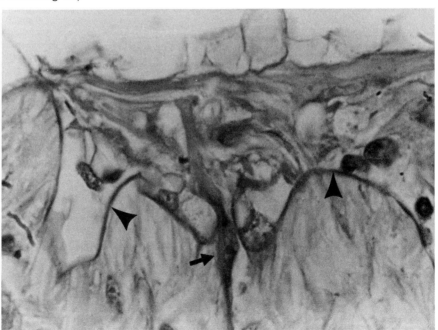

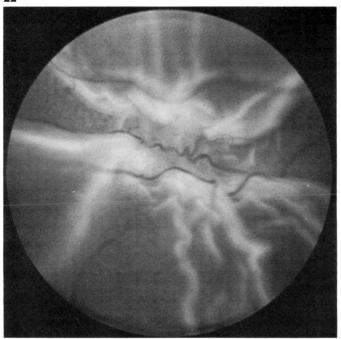

FIG. 2-12. Clinical appearance of fixed fold caused by pre-retinal proliferation. The retinal fold is concave toward the pupil.

FIG. 2-13. Fixed folds of outer retina caused by contraction of a membrane (*arrows*) on the outer retinal surface. Note folds in the external nuclear layer. (H & E × 16.) (Yanoff M, Fine BS: *Ocular Pathology, A Text and Atlas.* Hagerstown, Harper & Row, 1975)

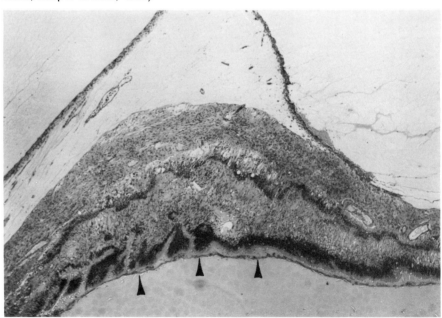

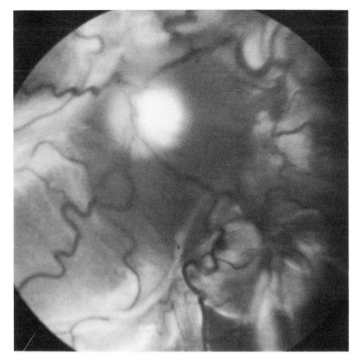

FIG. 2-14 Clinical appearance of massive periretinal proliferation largely caused by subretinal proliferations. (Yanoff M, Fine BS: *Ocular Pathology, A Text and Atlas.* Hagerstown, Harper & Row, 1975)

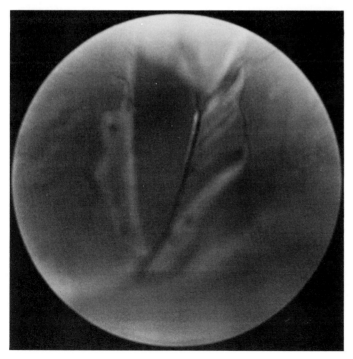

FIG. 2-15. Flap tear with posteriorly rolled edges. Notice bridging vessel.

membranes can cause equatorial traction folds and/or fixed folds.[15] Both glial and pigment epithelial cells can proliferate on the inner (Figs. 2-10, 2-11, 2-12) and outer retinal surfaces (Figs. 2-13, 2-14), causing fixed folds and/or irregular retinal folding.[3, 15, 16, 33, 35, 36]

Ten per cent of detached retinas have signs of periretinal proliferation, e.g., fixed folds, equatorial traction, or tears with posteriorly rolled edges (Fig. 2-15).[7, 28] Fortunately, only 25 per cent of these progress to massive periretinal proliferation.[28]

INTRAOCULAR PRESSURE

In eyes with rhegmatogenous retinal detachment, the intraocular pressure usually decreases in proportion to the extent and duration of the detachment.[4, 14] Fluorescein and tonographic studies have shown that this relative hypotony is caused by decreased aqueous secretion.[4, 14, 29]

In some cases, however, the intraocular pressure in an eye with retinal detachment may be elevated because of decreased aqueous outflow. The detachment in most of these eyes is of long duration. Because numerous small clumps of pigmented cells ("tobacco dust") are often found in the vitreous cavity and anterior chamber of eyes with longstanding detachment, it is postulated that the accumulation of these cells in the trabecular meshwork blocks aqueous outflow.[18, 32] The pressure and the outflow facility usually return to normal after the retinal detachment has been repaired.[32] It is important to remember that rhegmatogenous retinal detachment can cause increased intraocular pressure. If the detachment is not detected, the patient may be mistakenly treated for glaucoma or uveitis.

REFERENCES

1. **Benson WE, Nantawan P, Morse PH:** Characteristics and prognosis of retinal detachments with demarcation lines. Am J Ophthalmol 84:641, 1977
2. **Clarkson JG, Green WR, Massof D:** A histopathologic review of 168 cases of preretinal membrane. Am J Ophthalmol 84:1, 1977
3. **Constable IJ, Tolentino FI, Donovan RH, Schepens CL:** Clinico-pathologic correlation of vitreous membranes. In Pruett RC, Regan CDJ (eds): Retina Congress. New York, Appleton-Century-Crofts, 1974, pp 245–257
4. **Dobbie JG:** A study of the intraocular fluid dynamics in retinal detachment. Arch Ophthalmol 69:159, 1963
5. **Godtfredsen E:** Investigations into hyaluronic acid and hyaluronidase in the subretinal fluid in retinal detachment, partly due to ruptures and partly secondary to malignant choroidal melanoma. Br J Ophthalmol 33:721, 1949
6. **Hamasaki EI, Machemer R, Norton EWD:** Experimental retinal detachment in the owl monkey. 6. The electroretinogram of the detached and reattached retina. Albrecht von Graefes Arch Klin Ophthalmol 177:212, 1969
7. **Havener WH:** Massive vitreous retraction. Ophthalmol Surg 4:22, 1973
8. **Hogan MJ, Zimmerman LE:** Ophthalmic Pathology. Philadelphia, WB Saunders, 1962, pp 549–568
9. **Kaufman PL, Podos SM:** The subretinal fluid in primary rhegmatogenous retinal detachment. Surv Ophthalmol 18:100, 1973
10. **Kross AJ, Machemer R:** Experimental retinal detachment in the owl monkey. 3. Electron microscopy of the retina and pigment epithelium. Am J Ophthalmol 66:410, 1968

11. **Kroll AJ, Machemer R:** Experimental detachment and reattachment in the rhesus monkey: electron microscopic comparison of rods and cones. Am J Ophthalmol 68:58, 1969

12. **Kroll AJ, Machemer R:** Experimental retinal detachment in the owl monkey. 5. Electron microscopy of the reattached retina. Am J Ophthalmol 67:117, 1969

13. **Kroll AJ, Machemer R:** Experimental retinal detachment in the owl monkey. 8. Photoreceptor protein renewal in early retinal reattachment. Am J Ophthalmol 72:356, 1971

14. **Langham ME, Regan CDJ:** Circulatory changes associated with the onset of primary retinal detachment. Arch Ophthalmol 81:820, 1969

15. **Laqua H, Machemer R:** Clinico-pathological correlation in massive periretinal proliferation. Am J Ophthalmol 80:913, 1975

16. **Laqua H, Machemer R:** Glial cell proliferation in retinal detachment (massive periretinal proliferation). Am J Ophthalmol 80:602, 1975

17. **Lobes LA:** The electro-oculogram in human retinal detachment. Br J Ophthalmol 62:223, 1978

18. **Linner E:** Intraocular pressure in retinal detachment. Arch Ophthalmol [Suppl] 84:101, 1966

19. **Machemer R:** Experimental retinal detachment in the owl monkey. 2. Histology of the retina and pigment epithelium. Am J Ophthalmol 66:396, 1968

20. **Machemer R:** Experimental retinal detachment in the owl monkey. 4. The reattached retina. Am J Ophthalmol 66:1075, 1968

21. **Machemer R:** Pathogenesis and classification of massive periretinal proliferation. Br J Ophthalmol 62:737, 1978

22. **Machemer R, Buettner H:** Experimental retinal detachment in the owl monkey. 9. Radioautographic study of protein metabolism. Am J Ophthalmol 73:337, 1972

23. **Machemer R, Kroll AJ:** Experimental retinal detachment in the owl monkey. 7. Photoreceptor protein renewal in normal and detached retina. Am J Ophthalmol 71:690, 1971

24. **Machemer R, Laqua H:** Pigment epithelial proliferation in retinal detachment (massive periretinal proliferation). Am J Ophthalmol 80:1, 1975

25. **Machemer R, Norton EWD:** Experimental retinal detachment in the owl monkey. 1. Methods of production and clinical picture. Am J Ophthalmol 66:388, 1968

26. **Machemer R, Van Horn D, Aaberg TM:** Pigment epithelial proliferation in human retinal detachment with massive periretinal proliferation. Am J Ophthalmol 85:181, 1978

27. **Mandelcorn M, Machemer R, Fineberg E, Hersh SB:** Proliferation and metaplasia of intravitreal retinal pigment epithelial cell autotransplants. Am J Ophthalmol 80:227, 1975

28. **Morse PH:** Fixed retinal star folds in retinal detachment. Am J Ophthalmol 77:760, 1974

29. **Moses RA, Becker B:** Clinical tonography: the scleral rigidity factor. Am J Ophthalmol 45:196, 1958

30. **Mueller-Jensen K, Machemer R, Azarnia R:** Autotransplantation of retinal pigment epithelium in intravitreal diffusion chambers. Am J Ophthalmol 80:530, 1975

31. **Rosen E:** A photographic investigation of simple retinal detachment. Trans Ophthalmol Soc UK 88:331, 1968

32. **Schwartz A:** Chronic open-angle glaucoma secondary to rhegmatogenous retinal detachment. Am J Ophthalmol 75:205, 1973

33. **Smith TR:** Pathologic findings after retinal surgery. In Schepens CL (ed): Importance of the Vitreous Body in Retinal Surgery with Special Emphasis on Reoperations. St. Louis, CV Mosby, 1960, pp 61–75

34. **Sweeney DB, Karlin DB, Balazs E:** In Schepens CL, Regan CDJ (eds): Controversial Aspects of the Management of Retinal Detachment. Boston, Little, Brown, 1965, pp 316

35. **Teng CC:** Discussion of Smith TR: Pathologic findings after retinal surgery. In Schepens CL (ed): Importance of the Vitreous Body in Retinal Surgery with Special Emphasis on Reoperations. St. Louis, CV Mosby, 1960, pp 76–91

36. **Van Horn DL, Aaberg TM, Machemer R, Fenzl R:** Glial cell proliferation in human retinal detachment with massive periretinal proliferation. Am J Ophthalmol 84:383, 1977

37. **Yanoff M, Fine BS:** Ocular Pathology. Hagerstown, Harper & Row, 1975, pp 455–562

3

PREDISPOSING
CONDITIONS

Chapter 1 discussed the basic mechanism of primary or spontaneous rhegmatogenous retinal detachment. This chapter will discuss specific events and conditions which predispose to retinal breaks and subsequent detachment.

LATTICE DEGENERATION

Lattice degeneration is a condition of the peripheral retina characterized by thinning of the inner retinal layers and liquefaction of the overlying vitreous (Fig. 3-1A). Vitreous adhesions surround the characteristically elliptical areas of degeneration, which may be marked by a criss-crossing lattice work of white lines (hyalinized blood vessels).[63] In some cases,[63] glial cells proliferate along the vitreal surface. In pigmented lattice (Fig. 3-1B), retinal pigment epithelial cells proliferate into the retina. A typical area of lattice degeneration parallels the ora serrata. Less common is radial lattice, which parallels retinal blood vessels (Fig. 3-2). Lattice is found in 6 to 7 per cent of the population and is bilateral in 33 per cent of affected persons.[11] It is more common in myopic than in hyperopic eyes,[11] and its incidence rises as the axial length of the eye increases.[39] In 31 per cent of affected patients, atrophic round holes are present within the areas of degeneration.[13]

Lattice is the direct cause of 21 per cent of all retinal detachments[8] and is present in 41 per cent.[3] In 30 to 45 per cent of cases, the detachment is caused by atrophic holes in the lattice.[8, 13] Seventy per cent of such detachments are seen in myopic eyes and 70 per cent occur in patients younger than 40 years of age.[8, 67] Demarcation lines are common in these slowly progressing detachments, which have a surgical success rate of 98 to 100 per cent.[8, 67] In 55 to 70 per cent of cases, the detachment is caused by a tear beginning posterior to or at the end of a patch of lattice.[8, 13] Ninety per cent of these detachments are in patients 50 years of age or older, and only 43 per cent of the affected eyes are myopic.[8] The detachments progress more rapidly than do those arising from atrophic holes within lattice. Demarcation lines are not present. Ninety per cent can be successfully repaired.[8]

MYOPIA

High myopes are particularly prone to retinal detachment. Böhringer[9] found that the lifetime risk of retinal detachment for a person with myopia greater than 5 diopters who lives to the age of 60 is 2.4 per cent as compared to a 0.06 per cent risk for an emmetrope who reaches the age of 60. Myopes have 42 per

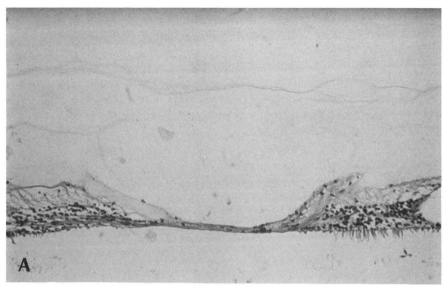

FIG. 3-1. (*A*) Lattice degeneration. Notice thinning of the inner retinal layers and liquefaction of the overlying vitreous. (H & E × 10. A.F.I.P. Accession No. 1319686). (*B*) Pigmented lattice degeneration with lattice work of hyalinized retinal blood vessels. At the right end of the lattice, a crescentic tear (*arrows*) is present.

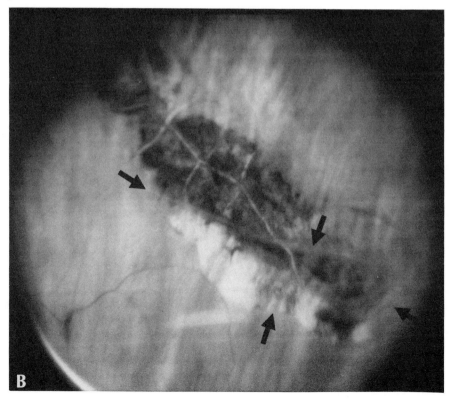

cent of all retinal detachments,[3] but they make up only 10 per cent of the population at large.[9] Moreover, myopes with a refractive error of greater than 8 diopters account for 10 per cent of all retinal detachments,[3] though they comprise only 1 per cent of the general population.[9]

Myopia predisposes to retinal detachment for three reasons. First, myopic eyes have an increased incidence of lattice degeneration.[11] Second, they have a higher incidence of posterior vitreous detachment.[35] Third, the thin retina of a myopic eye is prone to develop retinal breaks. Indeed, 18 per cent of eyes with 6 or more diopters of myopia have full-thickness retinal breaks,[34] as compared to a 7 per cent incidence for the population at large.

APHAKIA

Cataract extraction greatly increases the chances that a patient will develop retinal detachment. Approximately 2 to 5 per cent of patients undergoing cataract surgery will have a subsequent retinal detachment,[57] as opposed to 0.05 per cent among the phakic population.[9, 28, 60] Intracapsular and extracapsular extractions have substantially the same incidence of subsequent detachment.[33] If vitreous has been lost during the cataract extraction, the incidence of detachment increases to 7 per cent.[33, 71] Of high myopes undergoing cataract surgery, 6 to 8 per cent will later develop retinal detachment.[4, 61] One study[54] has shown that myopes of greater than 10.00 diopters have a 40 per cent likelihood of retinal detachment following cataract extraction. Fifty per cent of aphakic retinal detachments occur within 1 year after cataract surgery.[3]

Patients who have had retinal detachment surgery are at some risk of redetachment if the cataract is subsequently removed. Ackerman[2] studied 73 eyes which had had retinal detachment surgery before undergoing cataract extraction. In three eyes (7 per cent), the retina subsequently redetached. All three detachments occurred within 1 month of the cataract operation, and two of the three developed inoperable massive periretinal proliferation.

The incidence of bilateral retinal detachment is much higher in aphakic than in phakic eyes. Campbell[14] studied the second eye of patients who had had a retinal detachment (phakic or aphakic) in the first eye. In all of these cases, the second eye was phakic at the outset of the study. Forty-one per cent of the second eyes developed retinal detachment after subsequent cataract extraction. He reported the same incidence of aphakic retinal detachment in the second eye, whether the retinal detachment in the first eye had been phakic or aphakic. Benson and colleagues[6] studied the second eyes of patients who presented with aphakic retinal detachment in the first eye. They found that a retinal detachment developed in 7 per cent of the second eyes which never underwent cataract extraction. This figure rose to 26 per cent if the cataract in the second eye was removed. In other words, even if the cataract is not removed in the second eye, the patient is at high risk of retinal detachment. Removing the cataract increases the risk approximately fourfold.

Compared to phakic retinal detachments, aphakic detachments are more commonly total (38 per cent versus 20 per cent); the macula is more often detached (83 per cent versus 65 per cent); and the retina more often has fixed folds, a sign of early massive periretinal proliferation (55 per cent versus 39 per cent).[3] The typical aphakic retinal detachment is caused by flap tears along the posterior vitreous base or small tears at the end of meridional folds. Superotemporal breaks predominate, as they do in phakic retinal detachment, but the incidence of superonasal breaks is somewhat higher in aphakic detachments.[20, 45, 52] No retinal breaks can be found in many more aphakic detachments (7 to 16 per cent) than in phakic detachments (2 to 4 per cent).[3, 24, 45]

The high incidence of retinal detachment in aphakic eyes is probably related to the high frequency of posterior vitreous detachment after cataract extraction.[30] Experimental evidence indicates that liquefaction and collapse of the vitreous body result from the diffusion of hyaluronic acid from the eye following the removal of the lens.[47] It was originally hoped that phacoemulsification would have a lower rate of subsequent retinal detachment because it can leave the posterior capsule intact. Unfortunately, the frequently required capsulotomy negates this theoretical advantage.[70, 72, 74] A similar hope was raised following the introduction of intraocular lenses. Early statistics indicate that this procedure does not reduce the incidence of postoperative detachment either.[36, 76] The rate of successful reattachment of the retina following these procedures is approximately the same as that following intracapsular cataract extraction (about 90 per cent),[74] but the final visual acuities are worse.[37]

Since aphakic retinal detachments are associated with a high incidence of periretinal proliferation, and since they have tiny breaks which may be missed on clinical examination, encircling procedures should be used in their treatment.

GLAUCOMA

There may be a genetic relationship between chronic open angle glaucoma and retinal detachment. A study of fellow eyes in patients who had unilateral retinal detachment—but did not have open angle glaucoma—found a significant percentage of decreased aqueous outflow facility, large cup/disc ratio, and marked elevation of intraocular pressure following administration of topical steroids.[59] Moreover, eyes with open angle glaucoma are prone to develop retinal detachment. Clinical studies[5, 41, 51] have reported that 4 to 7 per cent of patients with retinal detachment have chronic open angle glaucoma, whereas less than 1 per cent of the general population have this condition.[51]

It has been suggested that the miotic drugs used in glaucoma therapy can cause retinal detachment. There have been 120 cases reported of retinal detachment in glaucoma patients being treated with parasympathomimetics or anticholinesterases.[1, 29, 49, 22, 29, 42, 48] However, because there are thousands of patients who have used miotic drugs without developing a retinal detachment, this small number of cases is not sufficient evidence to prove that miotics cause retinal detachment.

Because glaucoma patients are more likely to develop retinal detachment than the population at large, they should have a careful peripheral retinal examination at regular intervals. Should they experience a sudden uniocular decrease in intraocular pressure, or should they have a sudden decrease in visual field despite adequate glaucoma control,[56] retinal detachment should be suspected and a dilated fundus examination should be performed.

TRAUMA

BLUNT TRAUMA

Blunt trauma or ocular contusion is a non-penetrating direct injury to the eye. It can cause various kinds of retinal breaks which may lead to detachment. Blunt trauma is the leading cause of retinal detachment in children and adolescents.[16, 75] Eighty-seven per cent of affected patients are males.[16]

Blunt trauma compresses the eye along its anterior-posterior diameter and expands it in the equatorial plane. Since the vitreous body is relatively elastic, slow compression of the eye has no deleterious effect on the retina. However, when the eye is rapidly compressed, the vitreous does not have sufficient time to stretch and there is resultant severe traction at the vitreous base.[73] This traction is usually strongest at the posterior border of the vitreous base and results in a linear tear in that area.[16] If the traction is strongest along the anterior border, the nonpigmented epithelium of the pars plana is torn.[65]

Strong traction along both the anterior and posterior borders of the vitreous base can tear the entire vitreous base away from the retina (avulsion of the vitreous base), generally tearing both the posterior retina and the pars plana in the process. This finding is pathognomonic of ocular contusion.[16]

The most common retinal tears resulting from blunt trauma are linear tears along the posterior border of the vitreous base and dialyses (separation of the retina from the nonpigmented epithelium of the pars plana at the ora serrata) (Fig. 1-10). The most common location for both kinds of tears was found to be superonasal in one large series[16] and inferotemporal in another.[27] Detachments due to dialysis characteristically progress very slowly and often bear the signs of longstanding detachment: demarcation lines and/or intraretinal cysts.[27] The interval between the trauma and the diagnosis of the detachment exceeds 8 months in 50 per cent of the cases.[16] The prognosis for successful reattachment of a detachment due to dialysis is excellent,[27] unless a giant tear is involved (see chapter 8, Surgery of Complicated Cases).

Blunt trauma can also cause posterior breaks, though these are rarer sequelae of trauma than either dialyses or tears along the vitreous base. A posterior flap tear can occur if the vitreous is strongly adherent to a focal area of retina. A direct blow can cause retinal necrosis, which may give rise to irregular retinal breaks with ragged edges. Also, shock waves (contrecoup) from anterior trauma may cause a macular hole.

Most retinal breaks due to blunt trauma probably occur at the time of impact. In two studies, patients with traumatic hyphema underwent a careful retinal examination as soon as the media were clear.[58, 65] Either tears along the posterior vitreous base or dialyses were found in 4 to 18 per cent of the eyes. Posterior breaks were found in 4 per cent. Follow-up found no late tears.

There has been controversy over whether or not indirect trauma can cause retinal tears. It seems likely that sudden acceleration of the vitreous by a blow to the head could produce a retinal tear in an eye predisposed to retinal detachment (such as an eye with high myopia or lattice degeneration). However, a study of 247 patients who had suffered severe head trauma failed to reveal any retinal breaks.[19]

PENETRATING INJURIES

Twenty per cent of posterior segment penetrating injuries result in a retinal detachment.[50] Detachment is 4.5 times likelier if vitreous hemorrhage is present (40 per cent versus 5 per cent).[50] Late retinal breaks are usually caused by contraction of episcleral fibrovascular tissue proliferating into the intravitreal space from the entry site of the foreign body (Fig. 3-3). The tears are located away from the entry wound of the foreign body.[15, 43, 50] Vitrectomy is often required to repair the detachment,[7, 15] although the prognosis is not good (see chapter 8, Surgery of Complicated Cases).

PROLIFERATIVE RETINOPATHIES

DIABETES

In diabetes, retinal anoxia stimulates the proliferation of new blood vessels along which fibroglial tissue grows. Posterior vitreous detachment in nondiabetic eyes is characterized by a clean separation of the posterior cortical vitreous from the retina. In diabetics, however, the vitreous may be strongly adherent to areas of the retina or to the fibrovascular proliferations. Therefore, as the vitreous body slowly collapses and moves forward, there is traction on the posterior retina. The most common type of retinal detachment in diabetics is non-rhegmatogenous traction retinal detachment. In these cases, the retina characteristically has a smooth surface and is immobile. The detachment is concave toward the front of the eye and rarely extends to the ora serrata. In many cases, a small traction retinal detachment will remain unchanged over many years. In others, there is a relentless progression into the macula. In the most severe cases, the retina is detached from equator to equator.

It is rare for diabetics with proliferative retinopathy to develop a rhegmatogenous retinal detachment.[24, 66] The breaks found in these cases are usually oval and are adjacent to fibrovascular proliferations from the retina (Fig. 3-4). Vitreous hemorrhage or the proliferation itself may block the examiner's view of the hole. However, even if the break cannot be located, the differential diagnosis can be made because the retina is mobile and has the irregular corrugations which are characteristic of rhegmatogenous retinal detachment (see chapter 2, Pathophysiology). The detachment is convex toward the front of the eye and usually extends to the ora serrata. Because of the vitreous traction, these detachments spread quickly and are difficult to repair (see chapter 8).

BRANCH RETINAL VEIN OCCLUSION

Branch retinal vein occlusion is a rare cause of rhegmatogenous retinal detachment.[26, 38, 53, 77] As in proliferative diabetic retinopathy, the retinal anoxia stimulates the proliferation of new blood vessels, which may adhere to the posterior cortical vitreous. When the vitreous body collapses, traction on the neovascularization can tear a hole in the retina, and a rhegmatogenous retinal detachment may result (Fig. 3-5).

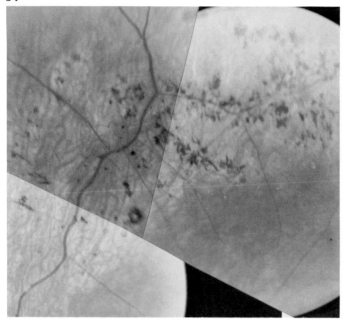

FIG. 3-2. Radial (or meridional) lattice degeneration which characteristically straddles retinal blood vessels and extends far posteriorly.

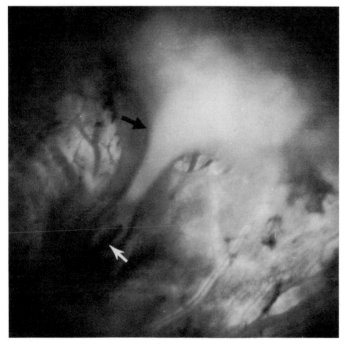

FIG. 3-3. Fibrovascular proliferation (*black arrow*) from the entry site of a foreign body to where it is now embedded (*white arrow*). Contraction of such tissue can cause retinal detachment.

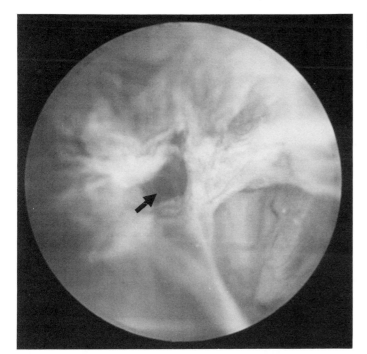

FIG. 3-4. Oval retinal break (*arrow*) caused by diabetic fibrovascular proliferations.

FIG. 3-5. (*A*) Rhegmatogenous retinal detachment caused by vitreous traction on neovascularization from branch retinal vein occlusion. Note rolled edge of the break. (*B*) Same break, closed by a scleral buckle.

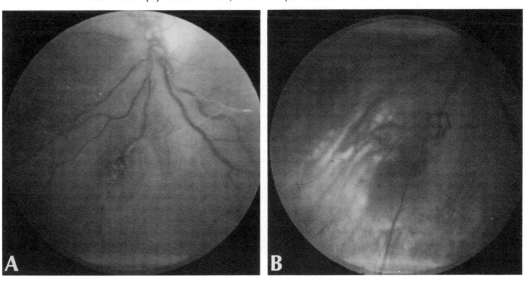

SICKLE CELL RETINOPATHY

Traction on proliferative fronds may cause rhegmatogenous retinal detachment. Anterior segment necrosis may complicate surgical repair.[55]

RETROLENTAL FIBROPLASIA

Rhegmatogenous retinal detachment is an uncommon late complication of cicatricial retrolental fibroplasia.[21, 64] Intravitreal proliferation of fibrovascular tissue may make it difficult to find the retinal breaks. In some cases, very posterior breaks are present.

INHERITED DISEASES

WAGNER'S SYNDROME (VITREORETINAL DEGENERATION)

The hallmark of Wagner's syndrome is an optically empty vitreous cavity traversed by bands and membranes (Fig. 3-6). Other findings which may be present are cataract, myopia, optic atrophy, choroidal and pigment epithelial atrophy, radial and circumferential lattice degeneration, peripheral retinoschisis, retinal detachment, and glaucoma.[27, 32, 40] The electroretinogram is subnormal. Stickler[62] described similar eye findings plus cleft palate and arthropathy. Wagner's syndrome is autosomal dominantly inherited. The lattice degeneration, retinoschisis, and vitreous membranes predispose to retinal detachments, which may be difficult to repair because the retinal breaks are often large, multiple, and at different levels.[31] Moreover, the vitreous membranes may prevent settling of the retina and sometimes necessitate vitrectomy.[10, 31] In the largest series reported, the surgical success rate was 68 per cent.[31]

CONGENITAL RETINOSCHISIS

In this sex-linked recessive condition (also called juvenile retinoschisis), the nerve fiber layer is separated from the other layers of the retina.[18] This results in a characteristic spokewheel "cystoid" macula (Fig. 3-7). In the periphery, especially inferotemporally, the nerve fiber layer may be elevated into the vitreous. Holes in this elevated "inner wall" (Fig. 3-8) are common but do not cause retinal detachment. The rarer "outer wall" holes, i.e., holes through the remaining retinal layers, can cause detachment. The prognosis for successful repair is good.

EHLERS-DANLOS SYNDROME

Myopia and retinal detachment may accompany this autosomal dominant condition in which collagen fibrils throughout the body are not organized into a strong supporting network.[68] Repair of retinal detachment is hazardous because the sclera, which is largely composed of collagen, does not hold sutures well. Also, fragile choroidal blood vessels bleed easily when drainage of subretinal fluid is attempted.[49]

FIG. 3-6. Vitreous band in Wagner's syndrome. Aside from band(s), the vitreous is optically empty.

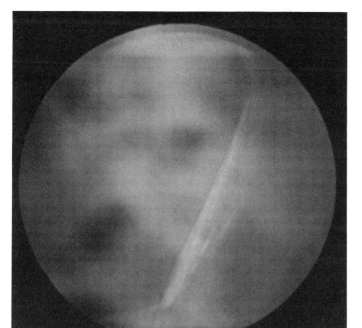

FIG. 3-7. Juvenile retinoschisis. Typical cystoid spoking pattern in fovea.

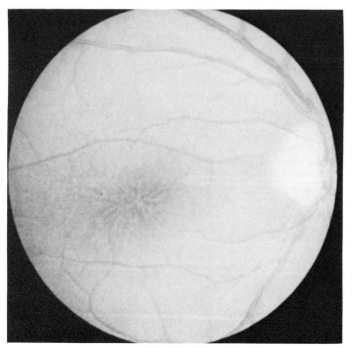

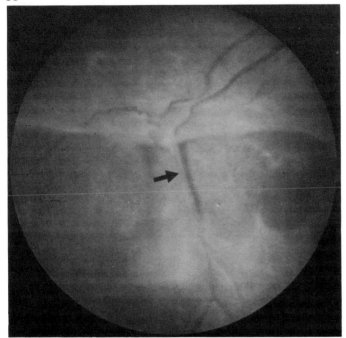

FIG. 3-8. Juvenile retinoschisis. Large hole in inner wall with bridging vessel (*arrow*).

GOLDMANN–FAVRE SYNDROME

This autosomal recessive ocular condition is characterized by cataract, peripheral and macular retinoschisis, retinitis pigmentosa-like retinal changes, radial lattice degeneration, and an optically empty vitreous cavity with vitreous membranes. The patients suffer from night blindness and progressive visual loss. The electroretinogram is severely depressed. As in Wagner's syndrome, retinal detachments may be difficult to repair.

MARFAN'S SYNDROME AND HOMOCYSTINURIA

In these conditions, high myopia and lattice degeneration are common and predispose to retinal detachment. Moreover, most patients have ectopia lentis. Removal of the lens is frequently complicated by vitreous loss, further increasing the chances of retinal detachment.

REFERENCES

1. **Ackerman AL:** Retinal detachments and miotic therapy. In Pruett RC, Regan CDJ (eds): Retina Congress. New York, Appleton-Century-Crofts, 1972, pp 533–539
2. **Ackerman AL, Seelenfreund MH, Freeman HM, Schepens CL:** Cataract extraction following retinal detachment surgery. Arch Ophthalmol 84:41, 1970
2a. **Alpar JJ:** Miotics and retinal detachment: A survey and case report. Ann Ophthalmol 35:395, 1979
3. **Ashrafzadeh MT, Schepens CL, Elzeneiny IH, Moura R, Morse P, Kraushar MF:** Aphakic and phakic retinal detachment. Arch Ophthalmol 89:476, 1973

4. **Barraquer J:** Surgery of the Anterior Segment of the Eye, Vol 1. New York, McGraw-Hill, 1964, p 289

4a. **Beasley H, Fraunfelder FT:** Retinal detachments and topical ocular miotics. Ophthalmology 86:95, 1979

5. **Becker B:** Discussion of retinal detachment and glaucoma by Smith JL. Trans Am Acad Ophthalmol Otolaryngol 67:731, 1963

6. **Benson WE, Grand MG, Okun E:** Aphakic retinal detachment. Arch Ophthalmol 93:245, 1975

7. **Benson WE, Machemer R:** Severe penetrating injuries treated with pars plana vitrectomy. Am J Ophthalmol 81:728, 1976

8. **Benson WE, Morse PH:** The prognosis of retinal detachment due to lattice degeneration. Ann Ophthalmol 10:1197, 1978

9. **Böhringer HR:** Statistisches zu Häufigheit und Risiko der Netzhautablösung. Ophthalmologica 131:331, 1956

10. **Brown GC, Tasman W:** Vitrectomy in Wagner's vitreoretinal degeneration. Am J Ophthalmol 86:485, 1978

11. **Byer N:** Clinical study of lattice degeneration of the retina. Trans Am Acad Ophthalmol Otolaryngol 69:1064, 1965

12. **Byer N:** The natural history of retinopathies of retinal detachment and preventive treatment. In Michaelson IC, Berman ER (eds): Causes and Prevention of Blindness. New York, Academic Press, 1972, pp 397–400

13. **Byer N:** Changes in and prognosis of lattice degeneration of the retina. Trans Am Acad Ophthalmol Otolaryngol 78:114, 1974

14. **Campbell CJ, Rittler MC:** Cataract extraction in the retinal detachment prone patient. Am J Ophthalmol 73:17, 1972

15. **Cox MS, Freeman HM:** Retinal detachment due to ocular penetration. Arch Ophthalmol 96:1354, 1978

16. **Cox MS, Schepens CL, Freeman HM:** Retinal detachment due to ocular contusion. Arch Ophthalmol 76:678, 1966

17. **Deutman AF:** Sex-linked jeuvenile retinoschisis. In The Hereditary Dystrophies of the Posterior Pole of the Eye. Assen, The Netherlands, CC Thomas, 1971, pp 48–99

18. **Deutman AF:** Genetics and retinal detachment. Mod Probl Ophthalmol 15:22, 1975

19. **Doden W, Stark N:** Retina and vitreous findings after serious indirect eye trauma. Klin Monatsbl Augenheilkd 164:32, 1974

20. **Everett WG, Katzin D:** Meridional distribution of retinal breaks in aphakic retinal detachment. Am J Ophthalmol 66:928, 1968

21. **Faris B, Brockhurst RJ:** Retrolental fibroplasia in the cicatricial stage: the complication of rhegmatogenous retinal detachment. Arch Ophthalmol 82:60, 1969

22. **Freilich DB, Seelenfreund MH:** Miotic drugs, glaucoma, and retinal detachment. Mod Probl Ophthalmol 15:318, 1975

23. **Funder W:** Das Schicksal der einseitig an Netzhautabhebung Erblinden. Klin Monatsbl Augenheilkd 129:330, 1956

23a. **Gragoudas ES, McMeel JW:** Treatment of rhegmatogenous retinal detachment secondary to proliferative diabetic retinopathy. Am J Ophthalmol 81:810, 1976

24. **Griffith RD, Ryan EA, Hilton GF:** Primary retinal detachments without apparent breaks. Am J Ophthalmol 81:420, 1976

25. **Schepens CL, Marden D:** Data on the natural history of retinal detachment. 61:213, 1966

26. **Gutman FA, Zagorra H:** The natural course of temporal branch retinal vein occlusion. Trans Am Acad Ophthalmol Otolaryngol 78:178, 1974

27. **Hagler WS, North AW:** Retinal dialysis and retinal detachment. Arch Ophthalmol 79:376, 1968

28. **Haut J, Massin M:** Fréquence des décollements de rétine dans la population française. Pourcentage des décollements bilateraux. Arch Ophtalmologie 35:533, 1975

29. **Heimann K, Kyrieleis E:** Retinal detachment during therapy with miotics. Klin Monatsbl Augenheilkd 156:98, 1970

30. **Heller MD, Straatsma BR, Foos RY:** Detachment of the posterior vitreous in phakic and aphakic eyes. Mod Probl Ophthalmol 10:23, 1972

31. **Hirose T, Lee KY, Schepens CL:** Wagner's hereditary vitreo-retinal degeneration and retinal detachment. Arch Ophthalmol 89:176, 1973

32. **Hughes WF Jr, Owens WC:** Extraction of senile cataract: a statistical comparison of various techniques and the importance of preoperative survey. Am J Ophthalmol 28:40, 1945

33. **Hughes WF Jr, Owens WC:** Post-operative complications of cataract extraction. Arch Ophthalmol 38:577, 1947

34. **Hyams SW, Neumann E, Friedman Z:** Myopia-Aphakia. II. Vitreous and peripheral retina. Br J Ophthalmol 59:483, 1975

35. **Jaffe NS:** Vitreous detachments. In The Vitreous in Clinical Ophthalmology. St. Louis, CV Mosby, 1969, pp 83–98

36. **Jaffe NS, Eichenbaum DM, Clayman HM, Light DS:** A comparison of 500 Binkhorst implants with 500 routine intracapsular cataract extractions. Am J Ophthalmol 85:24, 1978

37. **Johnston GP, Okun E, Boniuk I, Arribas N, Escoffery R:** Pseudophakic retinal detachment. Mod Probl Ophthalmol 18:499, 1977

38. **Joondeph HC, Goldberg MF:** Rhegmatogenous retinal detachment after tributary vein occlusion. Am J Ophthalmol 80:253, 1975

39. **Karlin DB, Curtin BJ:** Peripheral chorioretinal lesions and axial length of the myopic eye. Am J Ophthalmol 81:625, 1976

40. **Knobloch WH, Layer JM:** Clefting syndromes associated with retinal detachment. Am J Ophthalmol 73:517, 1972

41. **Kolker AE, Hetherington J Jr:** Becker and Shaffer's Diagnosis and Therapy of the Glaucomas, 3rd ed. St. Louis, CV Mosby, 1970, pp 247–248

42. **Kraushar MF, Podell DL:** "Miotic-induced" retinal detachment. In Pruett RC, Regan CDJ (eds): Retina Congress. New York, Appleton-Century-Crofts, 1972, pp 541–545

43. **Labelle P, Brunet M, Basmadjian G, Dumas J:** Retinal detachment following intra-ocular foreign body. Can J Ophthalmol 9:2, 1974

44. **Mandelcorn MS, Blankenship G, Machemer R:** Pars plana vitrectomy for the management of severe diabetic retinopathy. Am J Ophthalmol 81:561, 1976

45. **Norton EWD:** Retinal detachment in aphakia. Trans Am Ophthalmol Soc 61:770, 1963

46. **Optiz JM:** Ocular anomalies in malformation syndromes. Trans Am Ophthalmol Otolaryngol 76:1193, 1972

47. **Österlin S:** Vitreous changes after cataract extraction. In Freeman HM, Hirose T, Schepens CL (eds): Vitreous Surgery and Advances in Fundus Diagnosis and Treatment. New York, Appleton-Century-Crofts, 1977, pp 15–21

48. **Pape LG, Forbes M:** Retinal detachment and miotic therapy. Am J Ophthalmol 85:558, 1978

49. **Pemberton JW, Freeman HM, Schepens CL:** Familial retinal detachment and the Ehlers-Danlos Syndrome. Arch Ophthalmol 76:817, 1966

50. **Percival SPB:** Late complications from posterior segment intraocular foreign bodies. Br J Ophthalmol 56:462, 1972

51. **Phelps CD, Burton TC:** Glaucoma and retinal detachment. Arch Ophthalmol 95:418, 1977

52. **Phillips CI:** Distribution of breaks in aphakic and "senile" eyes with retinal aphakic detachment. Br J Ophthalmol 47:744, 1963

53. **Regenbogen L, Gode V, Feiler-Ofrey V, Stein R:** Retinal breaks secondary to vascular accidents. Am J Ophthalmol 84:187, 1977

54. **Ruben M, Rajpurohit P:** Distribution of myopia in aphakic retinal detachments. Br J Ophthalmol 60:517, 1976

55. **Ryan SJ, Goldberg MF:** Anterior segment ischemia following scleral buckling in sickle cell hemoglobinopathy.

56. **Sarin LK, Chessen GJ, McDonald PR:** The problem of retinal detachment in the presence of glaucoma. Am J Ophthalmol 56:908, 1973

57. **Scheie HG, Morse PH, Aminlari A:** Incidence of retinal detachment following cataract extraction. Arch Ophthalmol 89:293, 1973

58. **Sellors PJ, Mooney D:** Fundus changes after traumatic hyphaema. BR J Ophthalmol 57:600, 1973

59. **Shammas HF, Halasa AH, Faris BM:** Intraocular pressure, cup-disc ratio, and steroid responsiveness in retinal detachment. Arch Ophthalmol 94:1108, 1976

60. **Stein R, Feller-Ofry V, Ramano A:** The effect of treatment in the prevention of retinal detachments. In Machaelson IC, Berman ER (eds): Causes and Prevention of Blindness. New York, Academic Press, 1972, pp 409–410

61. **Stein R, Pinchas A, Treister G:** Prevention of retinal detachment by a circumferential barrage prior to lens extraction in high myopic eyes. Ophthalmologica 165:125, 1972

62. **Stickler GB, Belau PG, Farrell FJ, Jones JD, Pugh DG, Steinberg AG, Ward LE:** Hereditary progressive arthroophthalmopathy. Mayo Clin Proc 40:433, 1965

63. **Streeten BW, Bert M:** Retinal surface in lattice degeneration of the retina. Am J Ophthalmol 74:1201, 1972

64. **Tasman W:** Vitreoretinal changes in cicatricial retrolental fibroplasia. Trans Am Ophthalmol Soc 68:548, 1970

65. **Tasman W:** Peripheral retinal changes following blunt trauma. Ophthalmol Soc 70:190, 1972

66. **Tasman W:** Retinal detachment secondary to proliferative diabetic retinopathy. Arch Ophthalmol 87:286, 1972

67. **Tillery WV, Lucier AC:** Round atrophic holes in lattice degeneration—an important cause of phakic retinal detachment. Trans Am Acad Ophthalmol Otolaryngol 81:509, 1976

68. **Tolentino FI, Schepens CL, Freeman HM:** Ehlers-Danlos Syndrome. In Vitreoretinal Disorders, Diagnosis and Management. Philadelphia, WB Saunders, 1976, pp 278–281

69. **Törnquist R:** Bilateral retinal detachment. Acta Ophthalmol (Kbh) 41:126, 1963

70. **Troutman RC, Clahane AC, Emery JM, Fink AI, Kelman CD, Ryan SJ, Welsh R:** Cataract survey of the cataract-phacoemulsification committee. Trans Am Acad Ophthalmol Otolaryngol 79:178, 1975

71. **Vail D:** After-results of vitreous loss. Am J Ophthalmol 59:573, 1965

72. **Watzke RC:** (Letter to the editor): Retinal detachment following phacoemulsification. Ophthalmology 85:546, 1978

73. **Weidenthal DT, Schepens CL:** Peripheral fundus changes associated with ocular contusion. Am J Ophthalmol 62:465, 1966

74. **Wilkinson CP, Anderson LS, Little JH:** Retinal detachment following phacoemulsification. Ophthalmology 85:151, 1978

75. **Winslow R, Tasman W:** Juvenile rhegmatogenous retinal detachment. Trans Am Acad Ophthalmol Otolaryngol 85:607, 1978

76. **Worst JGF, Mosselman CD, Ludwig HHH:** The artificial lens: experience with 2000 lens implantations. Am Intraocular Implant Soc J 3:14, 1977

77. **Zauberman H:** Retinopathy of retinal detachment after major vascular occlusions. Br J Ophthalmol 52:117, 1968

4

HISTORY

The history of the diagnosis and management of retinal detachment begins, for all practical purposes, with the invention of the ophthalmoscope by von Helmholtz in 1851. He thereby provided not only the means for accurate clinical descriptions of retinal detachment but also an impetus for its cure.

Numerous incorrect theories of etiology and misguided attempts at treatment preceded the postulation of the rhegmatogenous theory by Leber and Gonin. In 1919, Gonin performed the first operation in which the goal was to cure the detachment by closing the breaks. The period between 1929 (when Gonin's procedure received acceptance) and 1935 was marked by advances in surgical technique. Major contributions in the modern period (1936 to the present) have been in instrumentation and technique.

THE EARLY PERIOD (1851–1918)

INSTRUMENTS FOR EXAMINATION

Shortly after the invention of the direct ophthalmoscope by von Helmholtz in 1851,[62] accurate clinical descriptions of retinal detachment were reported by von Graefe[59] and von Arlt.[58] In 1852, Ruete[47] introduced the monocular indirect ophthalmoscope. This instrument was later improved upon and became popular in Europe. In 1861, Giraud-Teulon[15] invented a binocular indirect ophthalmoscope. In 1900, Trantas,[56] with the aid of the direct ophthalmoscope, examined the anterior portion of the retina using his thumb to depress the sclera. Gullstrand's invention of the slit lamp in 1911 was another important advance.[21] In conjunction with either the pre-corneal lenses of Lemoine-Valois[57] or Hruby,[23] or with Koeppe's corneal contact lens,[26] the slit lamp provided a binocular view of the posterior portions of the eye.

INCORRECT THEORIES OF ETIOLOGY

Theory of Distension. It was soon recognized that retinal detachment was much more frequent in myopic than in emmetropic and hyperopic eyes. Von Graefe[61] proposed that the retina detached because it was less elastic than the choroid and the sclera, which stretched as the globe became larger (Fig. 4-1).

Theory of Hypotony. Because eyes with retinal detachment often have decreased intraocular pressure, and because many eyes which suffer vitreous loss during cataract surgery later develop retinal detachment, some physicians[18] hypothesized that a reduction of "vitreous pressure" induced detachment. They held that the formed vitreous gel, in its normal state, helped to counterbalance "hydrostatic pressure" exerted by the choroid.

Iwanoff[24] supplied histopathological evidence for this theory when he found vitreous liquefaction and posterior vitreous detachment in most eyes with retinal detachment. Supposedly, the liquid vitreous did not exert as much pressure as did the vitreous gel (Fig. 4-2).

Theory of Exudation. Recognizing that severe nephritis and toxemia of pregnancy—conditions in which generalized edema is common—are both causes of retinal detachment, certain ophthalmologists postulated that exudation of fluid from the choroid induced detachment (Fig. 4-3). We now know, of course, that the retinal detachment in these conditions is non-rhegmatogenous in nature and is reversible with treatment of the underlying disease state.

A variant of the exudation theory, taking into consideration the inflammation noted in many eyes with retinal detachment, proposed that the inflamed choroid exuded a highly albuminous fluid under the retina (Fig. 4-4*A*).[45] Osmotic pressure exerted by this exudate purportedly drew water from the vitreous through the retina, thereby elevating it from the choroid (Fig. 4-4*B*). Supporters of this theory felt that retinal breaks noted on clinical examination were secondary to the force of this exudative fluid. Since the edges of many tears were noted to be rolled outward, it seemed likely that fluid was passing from the subretinal space into the vitreous cavity.

ATTEMPTS AT TREATMENT

Since the main problem in retinal detachment appeared to be fluid under the retina, it is not surprising that the earliest attempted treatment was simple drainage of the fluid.[60] Very few cures resulted, as the fluid quickly reaccumulated postoperatively.

A different approach was taken by those who felt that retinal detachment was caused by exudation. These surgeons deliberately slashed holes in the retina to allow the subretinal fluid to pass into the vitreous.[60] The same tactic was tried by those who felt that the stiff retina would not reattach unless relaxing incisions were made.[55] Another futile attempt to counteract exudation was the injection of hypertonic (30 per cent) saline under the conjunctiva to draw out the subretinal fluid.

Some surgeons attempted to create scars between the retina and pigment epithelium to hold the retina in place.[11] Thermocautery and direct current electricity (galvanocautery) were two early treatment modalities. The treatment was not directed at retinal breaks but was randomly applied in the area of the detachment. Other surgeons tried to suture the retina to the choroid.[13] On histopathological examination, Müller[42] found vitreoretinal fibrous bands which he felt were pulling the retina forward and causing the detachment. His finding led Deutschmann[9] to postulate that the retina could be reattached only if the vitreous bands were sectioned. He introduced a fine knife into the vitreous and slashed backwards and forwards in an effort to sever them. The

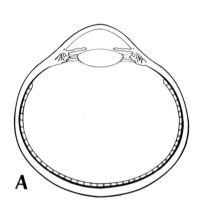

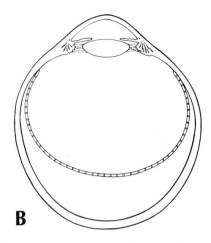

FIG. 4-1. Theory of distension. (*A*) Normal eye. (*B*) As the eye enlarges in high myopia the "less elastic" retina detaches.

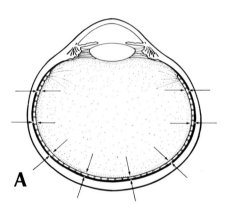

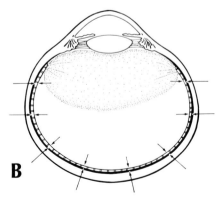

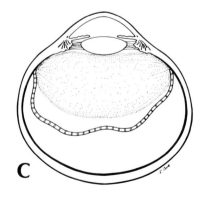

FIG. 4-2. Theory of hypotony. (*A*) Normal eye. "Vitreous pressure" balances "hydro-static choroidal pressure." (*B*) Posterior vitreous detachment. "Vitreous pressure" is reduced. (*C*) Resultant retinal detachment.

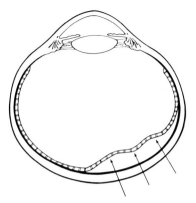

FIG. 4-3. Theory of exudation. An outpouring of fluid from the choroid elevates the retina.

FIG. 4-4. Theory of exudation. Diffusion variant. (*A*) The osmotic pressure of the protein-rich choroidal exudate draws water from the protein-poor vitreous through the retina. (*B*) Diffusion continues until the osmotic pressure is equal on both sides of the retina.

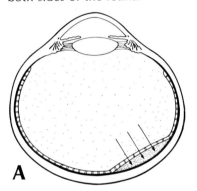

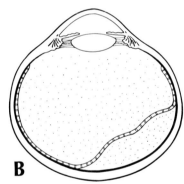

A

B

retinal tears which were sometimes produced in the process were not felt to be a complication. On the contrary, it was believed that the holes would help the retina to settle.

The theory of distension suggested another form of therapy. Since the retina was too short for the size of the globe, it seemed necessary to make the globe smaller. Müller[43] introduced the scleral resection operation in 1903. He excised a full-thickness wedge of sclera and then sewed the edges together.

THE GONIN ERA (1919–1935)

THE RHEGMATOGENOUS THEORY

Coccius[6] was the first to find retinal breaks on clinical examination, but deWecker[10] first suggested that they were the cause of what was then called spontaneous retinal detachment. He felt that liquid vitreous forced holes in the retina. Leber[29] found retinal breaks in 70 per cent of recent retinal detachments and noted that there was nearly always a retinal break in the area where the retinal detachment started. His own clinical and histopathological findings led him to conclude that vitreous traction, caused by degeneration and collapse of the vitreous body, tore holes in the retina. Liquefied vitreous passed through these holes and under the retina, causing the detachment.

It is apparent that at this point Leber understood the etiology of retinal detachment. In 1908, however, influenced more by histopathological than by clinical findings, he abandoned his initial theory in favor of an incorrect one.[20, 31] He now postulated that retinitis stimulated the growth of preretinal membranes which later contracted, tearing holes in the retina. He still recognized the importance of retinal breaks in the genesis of retinal detachment, but he now maintained that vitreous degeneration was secondary to the detachment, and not its precipitating event. It is apparent from Leber's drawings that his error stemmed from studying cases of retinal detachment with massive periretinal proliferation.

THE IGNIPUNCTURE (THERMOCAUTERY) OPERATION

Jules Gonin, the father of retinal detachment surgery, revived Leber's first theory,[12] stressing that contraction of the vitreous body tore holes in the retina. The tears occurred at sites of abnormal vitreoretinal adhesion caused by either a previous chorioretinitis or by chorioretinal degeneration. Once Gonin realized that the breaks found in retinal detachment were the cause of the detachment, he knew that a permanent cure depended on sealing them. In 1919, he performed the first operation designed to close the breaks.[17, 19] After careful localization of the break, he made a radial incision down to the choroid with a Graefe knife. The same knife was then used to drain the subretinal fluid. Next, a red-hot cautery was inserted 2 to 3 mm. into the wound and held in place for 2 to 3 seconds to insure that the retina had been directly cauterized (Fig. 4-5). It was not until 1929 that the world became convinced that Gonin's operation would cure retinal detachment.[19]

Gonin had achieved a miracle. Retinal detachment, which had previously been considered inoperable, now had a surgical success rate of 40 to 50 per cent. Gonin's two principles have remained the basis for all successful retinal detachment surgery. The first is that all breaks must be found. He emphasized careful clinical examination to this end. The second principle is that all breaks must be accurately localized so that they can be sealed by the treatment. Gonin recognized that a surgical failure meant either that the retinal break was not properly closed or that another break existed which had not yet been found. Once it was recognized that sealing the hole would cure a detachment, others quickly improved upon Gonin's original operation. Complications of his ignipuncture operation included intraocular hemorrhage and vitreous loss with retinal incarceration. Retinal folds often prevented reattachment of the retina. Fibrous ingrowth caused late redetachment. Another problem was that an essential part of the operation, exact localization of the break on the sclera, was extremely difficult. Because of the severe hypotony which followed removal of the cautery, only one puncture could be performed in a single operation. Therefore, if the localization were incorrect and the retinal break inadequately treated, a second operation became necessary. Furthermore, since only one break could be treated at a time, cases with multiple breaks required multiple operations.

EARLY IMPROVEMENTS ON IGNIPUNCTURE (1930–1933)

Guist's Operation (Multiple Trephination). Guist trephined out multiple plugs of sclera surrounding the retinal tear(s) and treated the bare choroid with a potassium hydroxide stick.[20] Once the subretinal fluid had been drained, chorioretinal scars formed and walled off the retinal break (Fig. 4-6).

Larsson's Operation (Surface Diathermy). When electric current flows in a resistive conductor such as the tissues of the eye, the heat generated causes localized coagulation. Larsson[27, 28] used this principle to surround the retinal break with a firm chorioretinal scar. He found that applications of diathermy (radiofrequency electric current) to full-thickness sclera coagulated the choroid (Fig. 4-7). Drainage of the subretinal fluid then brought the retina into contact with the treated choroid. If no tear could be found, he scattered treatment in the area which he felt had detached first.

Weve's Operation (Penetrating Diathermy). Weve improved upon Gonin's procedure by substituting penetrating diathermy for heat cautery.[64] A fine needle electrode introduced into the eye coagulated the choroid and the retina. Gonin's procedure allowed only a single application of cautery, whereas Weve's operation made multiple applications of treatment possible. His rate of success was therefore higher because his chances of sealing the break were better. Coagulation of the retina appeared as a white mark which could be observed with an ophthalmoscope and used as a guide in positioning the next penetration. Each time the needle was removed from the sclera, there was some drainage of subretinal fluid. The procedure was continued until the tear was completely surrounded by treatment. The major advantage of this proce-

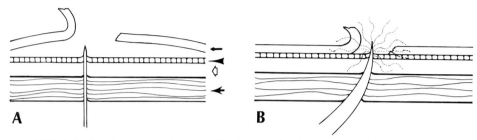

FIG. 4-5. Gonin's operation. (*A*) Drainage of subretinal fluid by a Graefe knife. Small arrow indicates the retina; arrowhead, the pigment epithelium; open arrow, the choroid; and large arrow, the sclera. (*B*) Coagulation of the choroid by thermocautery.

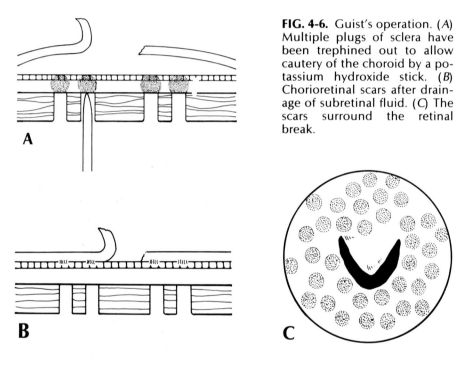

FIG. 4-6. Guist's operation. (*A*) Multiple plugs of sclera have been trephined out to allow cautery of the choroid by a potassium hydroxide stick. (*B*) Chorioretinal scars after drainage of subretinal fluid. (*C*) The scars surround the retinal break.

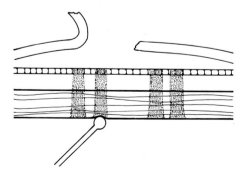

FIG. 4-7. Larsson's operation. Applications of full-thickness diathermy surround the break.

dure was that at the end of the procedure the retinal break was completely treated and no subretinal fluid was present. As in Gonin's operation, however, vitreous was occasionally lost and the punctures sometimes produced new retinal holes.

Šafář's Operation (Simultaneous Multiple Puncture). Šafář mounted fine needles on small conducting plates.[48,49] He inserted the needles around the break piercing the sclera, choroid, and pigment epithelium. No needles were removed until diathermy had been applied to all of the plates (Fig. 4-8). Therefore, there was neither premature drainage of subretinal fluid nor vitreous loss. When the needles were removed, the subretinal fluid slowly oozed out. This operation was popularized in the United States by Walker[63] and Pischel.

Lindner's Operation (Scleral Resection). In 1931, Lindner revived Müller's scleral resection operation, i.e., removal of a full-thickness strip of sclera.[36,37,38,39] The bare choroid was coagulated by potassium hydroxide (Fig. 4-9). This operation had two theoretical benefits: First, it reduced the volume of the eye so that the retina could more easily fall into place; and second, multiple holes could be treated. However, the operation was dangerous and difficult. Deep lamellar resection, a safer and easier variation, had been abandoned by Lindner as ineffectual, but Shapland[54] and Paufique[44] revived it as an improvement in the early 1950s (Fig. 4-10). They recognized that this procedure, in which a very thin layer of sclera was left over the choroid, had the additional benefit of causing a broad area of inflammation which could treat unseen retinal tears.

THE MODERN PERIOD

INSTRUMENTS FOR EXAMINATION

The current high rate of reattachment is due not only to improvements in surgical technique but also to improved methods of ocular examination. Two significant advances in fundus examination were made in the late 1940s. Charles Schepens' electrically illuminated binocular indirect ophthalmoscope is the most valuable instrument currently available for evaluation of the detached retina (see chapter 6, Fundus Examination). The Goldmann three-mirror lens permits stereoscopic slit lamp examination of almost the entire retina if the pupil can be widely dilated and if the ocular media are clear. It is especially useful for finding small breaks and for evaluating the vitreous.

INTRAVITREAL AIR INJECTION

In 1938, Rosengren[46] increased the rate of reattachment by injecting air into the vitreous to tamponade the retinal break after diathermy treatment and drainage of subretinal fluid. Postoperatively, the patient had to be positioned so that the air rose against the hole (Fig. 4-11). Using this technique, Rosengren was able to achieve successful reattachment in 76 per cent of his cases.[32]

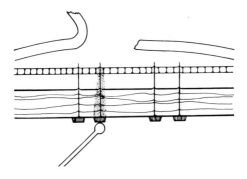

FIG. 4-8. Šafář's operation. Diathermy is applied to multiple fine needles which perforate the sclera, choroid, and pigment epithelium.

FIG. 4-9. Lindner's operation. (*A*) The bare choroid is cauterized by potassium hydroxide after a strip of full-thickness sclera has been removed. (*B*) The edges are sutured together. Shortening the sclera was the goal of the operation. The location of the resection did not necessarily correspond to the location of the break(s).

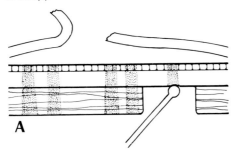

A

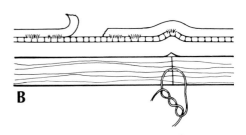

B

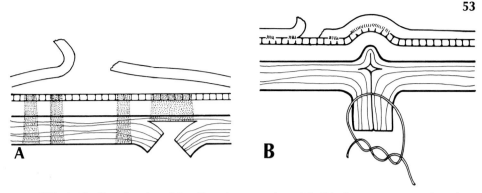

FIG. 4-10. Shapland and Paufique's operation. (*A*) Diathermy or potassium hydroxide coagulation is applied in the bed of the lamellar dissection. Diathermy surrounds the break. (*B*) The scleral flaps are closed, shortening the sclera.

FIG. 4-11. Rosengren's operation. (*A*) Applications of full-thickness diathermy to surround the break. (*B*) After drainage of the subretinal fluid, air is injected into the vitreous cavity. The patient is postioned so that air tamponades the break and pushes it toward the choroid.

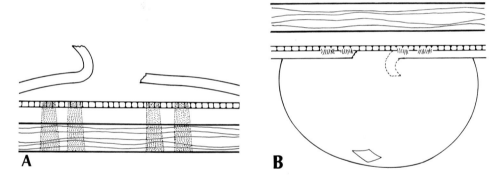

FIG. 4-12. Custodis' operation. (*A*) Applications of full-thickness diathermy to surround the break. Explant and sutures are positioned. Note vitreous traction (*arrow*). (*B*) The retinal break is closed by the indented ("buckled") sclera. The vitreous traction (*arrow*) is released.

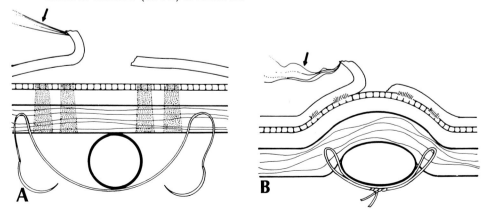

SCLERAL BUCKLING: EXPLANTS

In the history of retinal detachment surgery, scleral indentation ("buckling"), introduced by Ernst Custodis in 1953, is second in importance only to the contributions of Jules Gonin. Custodis called his procedure *plombenaufnähung,* literally, the sewing on of a seal.[7,8] He first treated all breaks with surface diathermy and then closed all breaks with a polyviol explant (the *plombe*) sewed to the sclera overlying the breaks. The indenting explant reduced vitreous traction and closed the break, allowing a firm chorioretinal scar to form (Fig. 4-12). Custodis emphasized that the explant must be large enough to close the entire retinal break, since a misplaced explant can keep the break open.

In addition to permanently reducing vitreous traction, Custodis' explant technique made drainage of subretinal fluid unnecessary in many cases. He found that even if the break remained open at the end of the operation a properly placed and correctly sized explant would result in successful reattachment of the retina. He was able to cure 84 per cent of his cases.

A major complication of Custodis' operation was that the surface diathermy caused scleral necrosis. If a reoperation became necessary, it was difficult to place sutures in the thinned sclera. Photocoagulation, invented by Meyer-Schwickerath,[41] eliminated this complication. The explant was placed, and, either immediately or 1 to 2 days later, the breaks were treated with photocoagulation.[2,14,22] Unfortunately, because xenon arc photocoagulation requires anesthesia, the patient was often subjected to 2 operative procedures. Moreover, successful treatment is dependent upon wide dilation of the pupil, which is often impossible immediately after a scleral buckling procedure.

Lincoff made the next major advances in explant technique by adapting cryotherapy for retinal surgery.[34] This was a more benign treatment than its predecessors, as it did not cause scleral necrosis. Lincoff also introduced a soft silicone sponge material[33] for use as an explant, and a spatula needle[35] for safe scleral surgery.

SCLERAL BUCKLING: IMPLANTS

One of the main problems in the use of diathermy was judging the effect on the choroid of applications made on full-thickness sclera. If the applications were not heavy enough, the retinal seal was inadequate. If the applications were too heavy, there was excessive scleral necrosis. Schepens, Black, and Clark[1,5,52] realized independently that Shapland's lamellar scleral resection could be used to thin the sclera so that the diathermy could be evenly and accurately applied to the choroid around the break. Then, when the scleral flaps were closed, the sclera was nearly restored to its original strength. Schepens[52] pioneered the use of implants in the scleral bed to reduce vitreous traction and to prevent posterior progression of the detachment. Originally, he buried polyethylene tubing at the posterior end of the most posterior break and drained the subretinal fluid. The implant was intended to act as a postoperative "dyke," preventing posterior leakage of subretinal fluid from any open anterior break. He later used implants made of solid silicone to completely close all retinal breaks (Fig. 4-13).[53] Another of Schepens' important contribu-

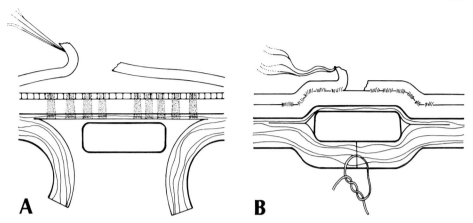

FIG. 4-13. Schepens' operation. (*A*) Diathermy is applied in the bed of the lamellar scleral dissection. Impant is positioned. (*B*) Sutured scleral flaps enclose the implant. Vitreous traction is reduced.

tions was the introduction of the encircling procedure to permanently reduce vitreous traction.[51, 52]

VITREOUS SURGERY

The first rational attempts at vitreous surgery were made by Cibis.[4] He realized that in "massive vitreous retraction" (massive periretinal proliferation), preretinal and vitreous membranes prevented settling of the retina. He slowly injected liquid silicone under these membranes to strip them from the retinal surface. Although many of these eyes had complications from the silicone or subsequent redetachment of the retina, many otherwise hopelessly lost eyes were saved by this procedure.[3]

Kasner performed the first planned vitrectomy in 1966.[25] Shortly thereafter, Robert Machemer[40] made a great advance in retinal surgery with the invention of the vitreous infusion suction cutter (VISC). Vitrectomy has increased the surgical success rate for retinal detachment with massive periretinal proliferation, for giant tear with rolled over retina, and for aphakic retinal detachment which will not settle because of vitreous caught in the cataract incision (see chapter 9, Postoperative Management).

REFERENCES

1. **Black G:** The role of the sclera in operations upon simple detachment of the retina. Trans Ophthalmol Soc UK 77:89, 1957
2. **Böke W:** Über die Kombination der Plombenaufnähung mit der Lichtokoagulation zur Behandlung der Netzhautablösung. Klin Monatsbl Augenheilkd 136:355, 1960
3. **Cibis PA:** Vitreoretinal Pathology and Surgery in Retinal Detachment. St. Louis, CV Mosby, 1965
4. **Cibis PA, Becker B, Okun E, Canaan S:** The use of liquid silicone in retinal detachment surgery. Arch Ophthalmol 68:590, 1962
5. **Clark G:** The importance and employment of diathermy in retinal detachment surgery of today. Arch Ophthalmol 60:251, 1958

6. **Coccius EA:** Uber die Anwendung des Augenspiegels nebst Angabe eines neuen Instrumentes. Leipzig, Immanuel Müller, 1853

7. **Custodis E:** Bedeutet die Plombenaufnähung auf die Sklera einen Fortschritt im der operativen Behandlung der Netzhautzblösung? Ber Dtsch Ophthalmol Ges 58:102, 1953

8. **Custodis E:** Scleral buckling without excision and with polyviol implant. In Schepens CL (ed): Importance of the Vitreous Body in Retina Surgery with Special Emphasis on Reoperations. St. Louis, CV Mosby, 1960, p 175

9. **Deutschmann R:** Ueber ein neues Heilverfahren bei Netzhautablösung. Beitr Augenheilkd 20:1, 1895

10. **de Wecker L, de Jaeger E:** Traité des maladies du fond de l'oeil et atlas d'ophtalmoscopie. Paris, 1870, pp 151–153

11. **de Wecker L, Masselon J:** Emploi de la galvanocaustique en chirurgie oculaire. Ann Oculist 87:39, 1882

12. **Dufour M, Gonin J:** Décollement rétinien. Encyclopédie Française d'Ophtalmologie. Paris, Doin, 1904

13. **Galezowski X:** Des Differentes variétés des décollements de la rétine et leur traitement. Recueil Ophtal 5:669, 1883–1884

14. **Girard LJ, McPerson AR:** Scleral buckling: full-thickness and circumferential, using silicone rubber rodding and photocoagulation. Arch Ophthalmol 67:409, 1962

15. **Giraud-Teulon M:** Note sur un nouvel ophthalmoscope binoculaire. Bull Acad Med (Paris) 26:510, 1860–1861

16. **Goldman H:** Slit-lamp examination of the vitreous and the fundus. Br J Ophthalmol 33:242, 1949

17. **Gonin J:** Guérisons opératoires des décollements rétiniens. Rev Gen Ophthalmol 37:295, 1923

18. **Gonin J:** Décollement idiopathique: Le processus pathogénique. In Le Décollement de la Rétine. Lausanne, Librairie Payot, 1934, pp 82–117

19. **Gonin J:** Le Traitment Operatoire. In Le Décollement de la Rétine. Lausanne, Librairie Payot, 1934, pp 138–246

20. **Guist G:** Fine neue Ablatiooperation. Z Augenheilkdl 74:232, 1931

21. **Gullstrand A:** Demonstration der Nernstspaltlampe. Ber Dtsch Ophthalmol Ges 37:374, 1911

22. **Höpping W:** Kombination von Lichtkoagulation mit operativen Verfahren bei Netzhautablösung. Ber Dtsch Ophthalmol Ges 64:512, 1961

23. **Hruby K:** Spaltlampenmikroskopie des hinteren Augenabschnittes ohne Kontaktglas. Klin Monatsbl Augenheilkd 108:195, 1942

24. **Iwanoff A:** Beitrage zur normalen und pathologischen Anatomie des Auges. I. Ablösung des Glaskorpers. Arch Ophthalmol 15:1–6, 1869

25. **Kasner D, Miller GF, Sever R, Norton EWD:** Surgical treatment of amyloidosis of the vitreous. Trans Am Acad Ophthalmol Otolaryngol 72:410, 1968

26. **Koeppe L:** Die Mikroskopie des lebenden Auges, Vol 2. Berlin, J Springer, 1921

27. **Larsson S:** Operative Behandlung von Netzhautablösung mit Elektro endothermie und Trepanation. Acta Ophthalmol 8:172, 1930

28. **Larsson S:** Electro-endothermy in detachment of the retina. Arch Ophthalmol 7:661, 1932

29. **Leber T:** Ueber die Entstehung der Netzhautablösung XIVth Vers. Ophthalmol Ges Heidelberg Bericht 1882, p 18

30. **Leber T:** Ueber die Enstehung der Netzhautablösung. Ber Dtsch Ophthalmol Ges 35:120, 1908

31. **Leber T:** Die Krankheiten der Netzhaut. In Graefe-Saemisch Handbuch der gesamten Augenheilkunde, Vol 7, part 2, 2nd ed. Leipzig, Wilheim Engelmann, 1916, 1374 pp

32. **Lehmann B:** Results of retinal detachment therapy at the eye clinic, Gothenburg 1936-1963. In Rosengren B (ed): Retinal Detachment Surgery. Acta Universitatis Gothoburgensis, 1966, pp 183–191

33. **Lincoff HA, Baras I, McLean J:** Modifications to the Custodis procedure for retinal detachment. Arch Ophthalmol 73:160, 1965

34. **Lincoff HA, McLean JM, Nano H:** Cryosurgical treatment of retinal detachment. Trans Am Acad Ophthalmol Otolaryngol 68:412, 1964

35. **Lincoff HA, Nano H:** A new needle for scleral surgery. Am J. Ophthalmol 60:146, 1965

36. **Lindner K:** Ein Beitrage zur Entstehung und Behandlung der idiopatischen und der traumatischen Netzhautabhebung. Albrecht von Graefes Arch Klin Ophthalmol 127:177, 1931

37. **Lindner K:** Unsere bisherigen Erfahrungen mit der Unterminierung methode bei Operation von Netzhautabhebungen. Ber Dtsch Ophthalmol Ges 49:83, 1932

38. **Lindner K:** Heilungversuche bein prognostisch ungünstigen Fallen von Netzhautabhebung. Z Augenheilkd 81:277–299, 1933

39. **Lindner K:** Shortening of the eyeball for detached retina. Arch Ophthalmol 42:635–645, 1949

40. **Machemer R, Buettner H, Norton EWD, Parel J-M:** Vitrectomy. A pars plana approach. Trans Am Acad Ophthalmol Otolaryngol 75:813, 1971

41. **Meyer-Schwickerath G:** Light-coagulation: a new method for the treatment and prevention of retinal detachment. XVII Concilium Ophthalmol 1:404, 1954

42. **Müller H:** Anatomische Beiträge zur Ophthalmologie. 7. Beschreibung einiger von Prof. v. Graefe exstirpieter Augäpfel. Graefes Arch Klin Ophthalmol 4(1): 363, 1858

43. **Müller L:** Eine neue operative Behandlung der Netzhautabhebung. Klin Monatsbl Augenheilkd 41:459, 1903

44. **Paufique L, Hugonnier R:** Traitement du décollement de la retine par la résection sclérale; technique personnelle, indications et résultats. Bull Soc Ophtalmol Franc 64:345, 1951

45. **Raehlmann E:** A critical comparison of Leber's theory of detachment of the retina, with the diffusion theory. Arch Ophthalmol (First Series) 23:92, 1894

46. **Rosengren B:** Über die Behandlung der Netzhautablösung mittelst diathermie und luftinjektionen in den Glaskörper. Acta Ophthalmol (Kbh) 16:3, 1938

47. **Ruete CGT:** Der Augenspiegel und das Optometer fur practische Aerzie. Göttingen, Dieterich, 1852

48. **Šafář K:** Behandlung der Netzhautabhebung mit multipler diathermischer Stichelung. Karger, Berlin, 1933

49. **Šafář K:** Detachment of the retina. Treatment with multiple diathermic puncture and its results. Arch Ophthalmol 11:933, 1934

50. **Schepens CL:** A new ophthalmoscope demonstration. Trans Am Acad Ophthalmol Otolaryngol 51:298, 1947

51. **Schepens CL:** Scleral buckling with circling element. Trans Am Acad Ophthalmol Otolaryngol 68:959, 1964

52. **Schepens CL, Okamura ID, Brockhurst RJ:** The scleral buckling procedures. 1. Surgical techniques and management. Arch Ophthalmol 58:797, 1957

53. **Schepens CL, Okamura ID, Brockhurst RJ, Regan CDJ:** Scleral buckling procedures. IV. Synthetic sutures and silicone implants. Arch Ophthalmol 64:868, 1960

54. **Shapland CD:** Scleral-resection-lamellar. Trans Ophthalmol Soc UK 71:29, 1951

55. **Sourdille G:** Une méthode de traitement de décollement de la rétine. Arch Ophthalmol 40:419, 1923

56. **Trantas A:** Moyens d'explorer par l'ophtalmoscope et par translucidité la partie antérieure du fond oculaire, le circle ciliaire y compris. Arch Ophtalmol 20:314, 1900

57. **Valois G, Lemoine P:** Ophtalmoscopie microscopique du fonde d'oeil vivant (sans verre de contact). Bull Soc Franç Ophtalmol 36:366, 1923

58. **von Arlt CF:** Die Krankheiten des Auges. 2:158, 1853

59. **von Graefe A:** Notiz über die Ablösungen der Netzhaut von der Chorioidea. Arch Ophthalmol 1:362, 1854

60. **von Graefe A:** Perforation von Abgelösten Netzhauten und Glaskorpermembranen. Arch Ophthalmol 9:85, 1863

61. **von Graefe A:** (Cited by Gonin J) Le Décollement de la Rétine. Lausanne, Librarie Payot, 1934, pp 82–84

62. **von Helmholtz H:** Beschreibung eines Augen-Spiegels zur untersuchung der Netzhaut im lebenden auge. (Description of an eye-mirror for the investigation of the retina in the living eye). Berlin, A Förstner, 1851

63. **Walker CB:** Retinal detachment. Technical observations and new devices for treatment with a specially arranged diathermy unit for general ophthalmic service. Am J Ophthalmol 17:1, 1934

64. **Weve H:** Zur Behandlung der Netzhautablösung mittels Diathermie Abhandlungen aus der Augenheilkunde. Heft. Berlin, 14 Karger, 1932

5

DIFFERENTIAL
DIAGNOSIS

Rhegmatogenous retinal detachment must be distinguished from exudative detachment, i.e., detachment caused by exudation of fluid from the choroid or retina in the absence of retinal breaks. If the underlying condition can be successfully treated, an exudative detachment will resolve. Rhegmatogenous detachment must also be differentiated from traction retinal detachment, which results from transvitreal traction on the retina, not from a retinal break. Traction detachments may not progress, but if the traction must be released, vitrectomy is the treatment of choice. Rhegmatogenous detachment can also be confused with entities which resemble it but which are not retinal detachments at all. Retinoschisis and choroidal detachment fall into this category. This chapter discusses the features which help the ophthalmologist to make the differential diagnosis.

RHEGMATOGENOUS RETINAL DETACHMENT

If no break can be found, the diagnosis of presumed rhegmatogenous retinal detachment can be made only after the conditions outlined in this chapter have been ruled out.

A history of light flashes and/or floaters followed by progressive visual field loss strongly suggests rhegmatogenous retinal detachment. It is also possible, however, for patients with malignant melanoma to notice light flashes[8] and for patients with cells in the vitreous from inflammatory conditions to complain of "floaters."

In rhegmatogenous detachment, the intraocular pressure is usually lower in the affected eye than in the fellow eye. Pigmented cells ("tobacco dust") are commonly present in the vitreous cavity and may be present in the anterior chamber. Detachments caused by flap or operculated tears frequently have associated vitreous hemorrhage. The detached retina undulates with eye movements. It is slightly opaque and often has a corrugated appearance. The subretinal fluid is clear and non-shifting. Irregular folds are common. Fixed folds, equatorial traction, and other signs of massive periretinal proliferation strongly suggest the diagnosis of rhegmatogenous detachment.

EXUDATIVE RETINAL DETACHMENT

An exudative detachment may be the direct result of a subretinal ocular condition which damages the retinal pigment epithelium, allowing choroidal fluid to pass into the subretinal space. Neoplasms and inflammatory diseases are the leading causes of such detachments. A hallmark of these detachments is "shifting fluid": the subretinal fluid responds to the force of gravity, detaching the area of the retina in which it accumulates. For example, when the patient is sitting, the inferior retina is detached. When the patient is then placed in the supine position, the fluid moves posteriorly in a matter of seconds or minutes, detaching the macula. Another characteristic of exudative detachments is the smoothness of the detached retina (Fig. 5-1), in contrast to the corrugated appearance seen in rhegmatogenous retinal detachment. Fixed folds are rarely, if ever, seen in exudative detachments (Fig. 5-2). Occasionally, the retina can be elevated enough in exudative detachments to be seen directly behind the lens. This rarely occurs in rhegmatogenous detachments. Specific etiologies of exudative detachment are discussed below.

NEOPLASMS

Choroidal malignant melanoma, metastatic carcinoma, and choroidal hemangioma are the most common neoplastic etiologies of exudative retinal detachment. The choroidal mass can usually be found by indirect ophthalmoscopy and confirmed by fluorescein angiography and ultrasonography. In addition to the mass, other differentiating features are shifting fluid, a biomicroscopically clear vitreous, and the absence of a retinal break.

In addition to causing retinal detachment, neoplasms can sometimes give the appearance of a detachment when none is present. The misnomer "solid retinal detachment" has been used to describe conditions in which both the sensory retina and the retina pigment epithelium are elevated by a choroidal or scleral mass. Such conditions may be mistaken for rhegmatogenous retinal detachment if the direct ophthalmoscope alone is used. With indirect ophthalmoscopy, such errors are rarely made, for stereopsis and the wide field of view identify the mass lesion (Fig. 5-3).

INFLAMMATORY DISEASES

Harada's Disease (Vogt-Koyanagi-Harada Syndrome)

Harada's disease is a bilateral uveitis usually seen in Blacks, Orientals, and darkly pigmented Caucasians. Systemic manifestations include headache, malaise, tinnitus, and nausea. Meningeal inflammation may cause stiff neck and cerebrospinal fluid pleocytosis. No sexual predilection is present. There may be associated papillitis. There are usually numerous inflammatory cells in the aqueous and vitreous. In early stages, multiple dome-shaped exudative retinal detachments are present. Later, they may coalesce into a large detachment with cloudy subretinal fluid. Fluorescein angiography reveals multiple areas of leakage through the retinal pigment epithelium. Most cases respond well to high doses of systemic corticosteroids.

Posterior Scleritis

Scleral inflammation can cause non-rhegmatogenous retinal detachment, usually with shifting, cloudy, subretinal fluid.[3] Most of the patients are

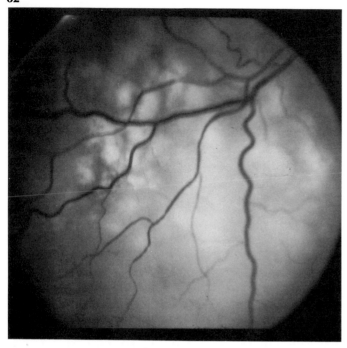

FIG. 5-1. Retinal detachment caused by metastatic carcinoma to the choroid. The retina is smooth. The mass can be seen under the detachment.

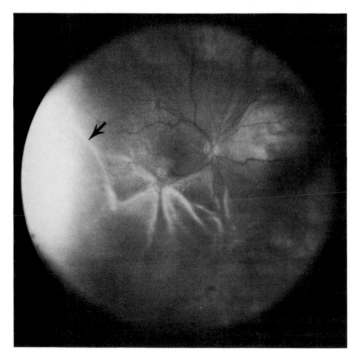

FIG. 5-2. Rhegmatogenous retinal detachment in an eye with coincidental malignant melanoma (nasal to optic nerve). Rhegmatogenous nature of detachment is shown by demarcation line (*arrow*) and fixed fold (inferotemporally). Shifting fluid was not present. The patient elected to have treatment of the melanoma by cobalt plaque. A scleral buckling procedure reattached the retina. (Courtesy of Jerry Shields, M.D. and Sheldon Kaplan, M.D.)

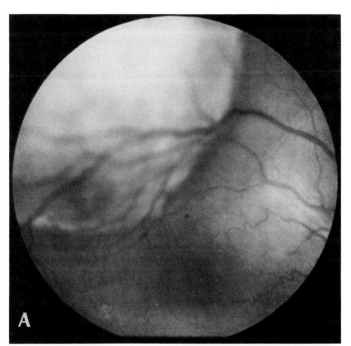

FIG. 5-3. "Solid" retinal detachment. (*A*) With direct ophthalmoscopy, the retinal elevation might be confused with rhegmatogenous detachment. (Courtesy of Jerry Shields, M.D.)

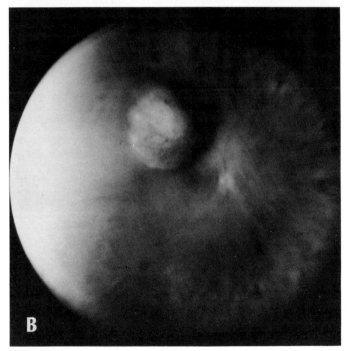

(*B*) Indirect ophthalmoscopy provides a wider field and stereopsis. It is apparent that a mass is elevating the retina. (Courtesy of Jerry Shields, M.D.)

women, and 50 per cent have rheumatoid arthritis. The condition is generally unilateral, with associated anterior scleritis and ocular, brow, or zygoma pain. If the inflammation is intense and localized, it can cause a posterior mass which indents the choroid and pigment epithelium. The mass can be found by indirect ophthalmoscopy. Ultrasonography differentiates it from choroidal neoplasms, which it may resemble. The ultrasonogram shows a thickened sclera with high internal reflectivity and retrobulbar edema.[3] Corticosteroids resolve the inflammation.

IDIOPATHIC CENTRAL SEROUS CHOROIDOPATHY (ICSC)

For unknown reasons, one or more small areas of the retinal pigment epithelium (RPE) lose their adhesion to Bruch's membrane, giving rise to RPE detachment(s). Choroidal fluid then passes through the RPE and accumulates under the sensory retina. In some cases of ICSC, multiple large RPE detachments allow passage of sufficient fluid to cause a bullous retinal detachment.[2, 7, 14] Most patients have bilateral evidence of ICSC. Some have bilateral bullous detachments. Others have a unilateral bullous detachment with either typical ICSC or asymptomatic RPE detachments in the other eye. ICSC is most common in white men between the ages of 30 and 50.

ICSC with bullous detachment can be confused with rhegmatogenous retinal detachment. In an ICSC detachment, there is shifting fluid, clear vitreous, and no retinal break—findings not characteristic of rhegmatogenous detachment. In addition, patients with ICSC do not complain of flashes or floaters. They usually notice blurring of the central before the peripheral vision. Finally, large RPE detachments in the posterior pole, characteristic of bullous ICSC, can be found by indirect ophthalmoscopy and confirmed by fluorescein angiography. They are usually effectively treated by argon laser photocoagulation.

OPTIC PIT

A congenital pit of the optic nerve head may cause a bullous retinal detachment.[9] There is rarely any difficulty in diagnosis, as the detachment usually extends in a tear-drop fashion from the abnormal optic disc.

TRACTION RETINAL DETACHMENT

Vitreous membranes caused by proliferative retinopathies or penetrating injuries can pull the sensory retina away from the pigment epithelium, causing a traction retinal detachment. The retina characteristically has a smooth surface and is immobile. The detachment is concave toward the front of the eye and rarely extends to the ora serrata (Fig. 5-4). In most cases, the causative vitreous membrane can be seen ophthalmoscopically or with the three-mirror lens. If the traction can be released by vitrectomy, the detachment may resolve. In some cases, traction tears the retina and causes a rhegmatogenous retinal detachment which is convex toward the front of the eye. The retina then becomes more mobile and has the irregular folds and corrugations characteristic of rhegmatogenous detachment. Treatment consists of a combination of vitrectomy to release the traction and a scleral buckling procedure to seal the break.

RETINOSCHISIS

SENILE RETINOSCHISIS

In senile retinoschisis, the retina is split into two layers ("walls") by a viscous substance presumed to be hyaluronic acid.[15] In typical retinoschisis, the split is in the outer plexiform layer; in reticular, in the nerve fiber layer. Retinoschisis may resemble rhegmatogenous retinal detachment, but several factors help the ophthalmologist to make the correct diagnosis. First of all, 70 per cent of the eyes are hyperopic. Moreover, retinoschisis is largely a temporal condition, inferotemporal in 70 per cent and superotemporal in 25 per cent of the affected eyes. In 50 to 80 per cent of the patients, it is bilateral.[1,4] The condition is usually asymptomatic. No tobacco dust or hemorrhage is present. The schisis cavity is dome-shaped with a smooth and thin inner wall which, on eye movements, may shake like jelly but does not undulate (Fig. 5-5). (Rhegmatogenous retinal detachment, of course, has a corrugated appearance and does undulate with eye movements). The outer wall of retinoschisis has a pocked or pitted appearance which can be identified, through the thin inner wall, with the aid of scleral depression. The retinal vessels are often sheathed. Prominent cystoid degeneration and "snowflakes" or "frosting" (footplates of Müller cells) (Fig. 5-6) are seen near the ora serrata. The absolute scotoma found on visual field testing helps to distinguish retinoschisis from rhegmatogenous retinal detachment, which causes a relative scotoma. Longstanding rhegmatogenous detachment without massive periretinal proliferation may be confused with senile retinoschisis. As the duration of the detachment increases, necrosis and dropout of retinal cells cause the retina to become thinner and more transparent (Fig. 2-5). It may then resemble the inner wall of a retinoschisis cavity. Findings often present in longstanding detachment but not found in retinoschisis are small full-thickness holes, intraretinal cysts, dialysis, depigmentation of the underlying retinal pigment epithelium, and demarcation lines (Figs. 2-5 and 2-7).

In addition to simulating detachment, as discussed above, senile retinoschisis can, in some cases, cause rhegmatogenous retinal detachment. Breaks in the outer wall (Fig. 5-7), with or without coexistent inner wall holes, can give rise to a detachment (Fig. 5-8), which must then be treated by the usual procedures. Retinoschisis is responsible for 3.2 per cent of all rhegmatogenous detachments.[11] Retinoschisis retinal detachments characteristically advance very slowly beyond the margins of the schisis cavity, and they sometimes have demarcation lines. In some retinoschisis detachments, the schisis cavity collapses. Then the combined detached retinal layers look very much like a typical rhegmatogenous detachment. If the examiner has not correctly diagnosed the detachment as secondary to retinoschisis, he may not locate the breaks. If a retinoschisis retinal detachment is suspected, the examiner should carefully search posteriorly, where outer wall holes are frequently found. The

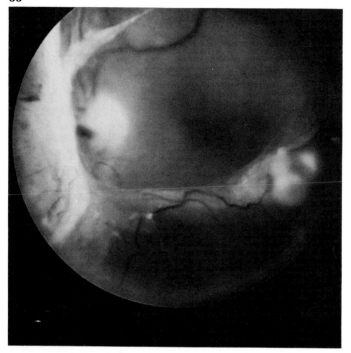

FIG. 5-4. Traction retinal detachment owing to proliferative diabetic retinopathy. The detached retina is smooth and is concave toward the pupil.

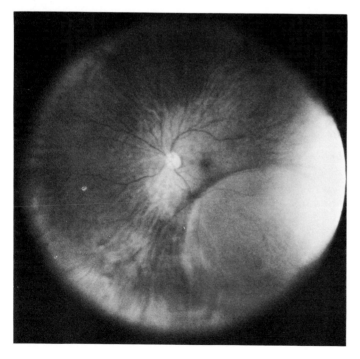

FIG. 5-5. Senile retinoschisis. Note the dome-shaped smooth inner wall and inferotemporal location. (Courtesy William Annesley, M.D.)

FIG. 5-6. Snowflake pattern seen near the ora serrata in senile retinoschisis.

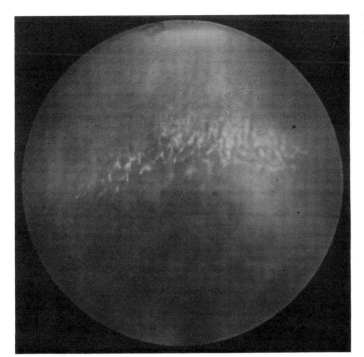

FIG. 5-7. Outer wall holes in senile retinoschisis.

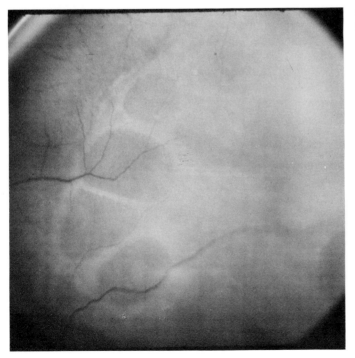

holes are generally round, with rolled edges (Fig. 5-8). The examiner can seek confirmation of the diagnosis in the patient's other eye; in 95 per cent of the cases of retinoschisis retinal detachment, the fellow eye has retinoschisis.[11]

JUVENILE RETINOSCHISIS

In this congenital, sex-linked, recessive condition, the retina is split in the nerve fiber layer.[5] Almost all affected eyes are hyperopic and have "cystoid" foveal changes (Fig. 3-7). The "cysts" are characteristically arranged in a spokelike configuration and do not stain with fluorescein. In half of the cases, retinoschisis is confined to the fovea. In the other half, the foveal changes are accompanied by an elevation of the inner retinal layer, in which large holes are commonly found (Fig. 3-8). This latter condition, most frequently present in the inferotemporal quadrant, might be confused with rhegmatogenous retinal detachment, but should not. Firstly, the retinoschisis does not extend to the ora serrata. Secondly, juvenile retinoschisis is a bilateral disease. Thirdly, the characteristic foveal "cystoid" configuration is not seen in any other condition except Goldmann-Favre disease.

CHOROIDAL DETACHMENT

A "choroidal detachment" (ciliochoroidal effusion) is an accumulation of fluid within the suprachoroidea, the outermost layer of the choroid, and within the supraciliaris, the outermost layer of the ciliary body. Technically, this condition is not a detachment because it involves swelling within a uveal layer, not a separation between the uvea and sclera. In actuality, however, the effusion separates most of the choroid and ciliary body from the sclera. Choroidal detachment is usually a sequela of ocular surgery, but it may also accompany ocular inflammatory conditions.[6, 12]

Choroidal detachments can be mistaken for rhegmatogenous retinal detachments, but they have several distinguishing features. They are orange-brown in color and have a more solid appearance than do retinal detachments because the retinal pigment epithelium and choroid are part of the elevated tissue. Hypotony, the elevation of the pars plana, and the absence of a retinal break also help to identify a choroidal detachment. Initially, a choroidal detachment has a smooth surface, but as it regresses, retinal folds may form (Fig. 5-9). Choroidal detachments jiggle on eye movements but do not undulate like rhegmatogenous retinal detachments.

Ultrasonography confirms the serous elevation of the choroid and pars plana, ruling out both neoplasms and retinal detachment. Choroidal detachments (unless hemorrhagic) transilluminate readily.

Choroidal detachment can appear in conjunction with rhegmatogenous retinal detachment (Fig. 5-10), posing an additional diagnostic problem. The coincidence of a brownish choroidal "mass" and a retinal detachment may lead to the mistaken diagnosis of malignant melanoma with associated serous detachment. Certain findings strongly suggest rhegmatogenous retinal detachment with associated choroidal detachment. One is severe hypotony; it is presumed that the retinal detachment causes hypotony, which then induces

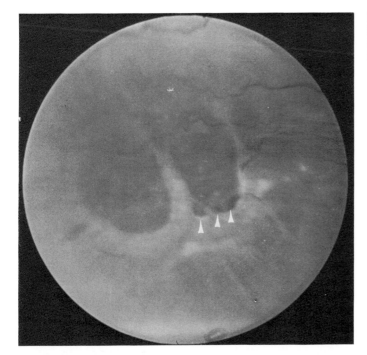

FIG. 5-8. Two large outer wall holes and three small inner wall holes (*arrowheads*) in retinoschisis–retinal detachment.

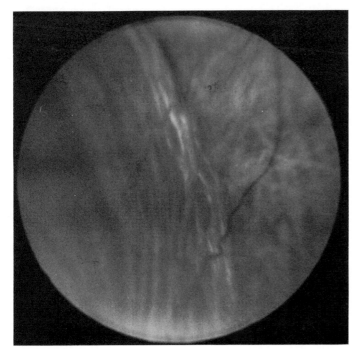

FIG. 5-9. Regressing choroidal detachment. Note the "solid" appearance, orange-brown color and retinal folds.

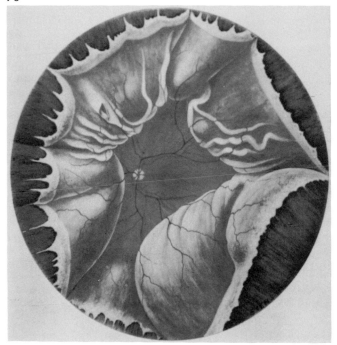

FIG. 5-10. Combined rhegmatogenous retinal detachment and choroidal detachment. The pars plana is significantly elevated. There is a superonasal retinal break. (Courtesy Dr. C. L. Schepens, Retina Foundation, Boston)

the choroidal detachment. When the ciliary body is detached, aqueous secretion is further decreased, lowering the intraocular pressure still more. The presence of a retinal break and pigmented cells in the aqueous and vitreous helps to identify the retinal detachment as rhegmatogenous. A choroidal detachment associated with rhegmatogenous detachment transilluminates, whereas a pigmented malignant melanoma does not. Finally, on ultrasonography, a choroidal detachment associated with rhegmatogenous detachment is acoustically empty, whereas a malignant melanoma is solid.

It is difficult to localize and treat retinal breaks through the suprachoroidal fluid. Therefore, the surgeon should try to resolve the choroidal detachment preoperatively. If systemic, topical, and periocular corticosteroids do not achieve this, the choroidal detachment must be drained during surgery. The prognosis for retinal reattachment is poor because there is a high incidence of massive periretinal proliferation (MPP).[10,13]

REFERENCES

1. **Ballantyne AJ, Michaelson IC:** Textbook of the Fundus of the Eye. Baltimore, Williams & Wilkins, 1970, pp 390–391
2. **Benson WE, Shields JA, Annesley WH Jr, Tasman W:** Idiopathic central serous retinopathy with bullous retinal detachment. (in preparation)
3. **Benson WE, Shields JA, Tasman W, Crandall AS:** Posterior scleritis. Arch Ophthalmol 97:1482, 1979
4. **Byer NE:** Clinical study of senile retinoschisis. Arch Ophthalmol 79:36, 1968
5. **Deutman AF:** The Hereditary Dystrophies of the Posterior Pole of the Eye. Assen, The Netherlands, CC Thomas, 1971, pp 48–99

6. **Fogle JA, Green WR:** Cilioretinal effusion. In Duane TD (ed): Clinical Ophthalmology Vol 4. Hagerstown, Harper & Row, 1978
7. **Gass JDM:** Bullous retinal detachment. An unusual manifestation of idiopathic central serous choroidopathy. Am J Ophthalmol 75:810, 1973
8. **Gass JDM:** Problems in the differential diagnosis of choroidal nevi and malignant melanomas. Am J Ophthalmol 83:299, 1977
9. **Gass JDM:** Stereoscopic Atlas of Macular Disease, 2nd ed. St. Louis, CV Mosby, 1977, pp 368–371
10. **Gottlieb F:** Combined choroidal and retinal detachment. Arch Ophthalmol 88:481, 1972
11. **Hagler WS, Woldoff HS:** Retinal detachment in relation to senile retinoschisis. Trans Am Acad Ophthalmol Otolaryngol 77:99, 1973
12. **Scheie HG, Morse PH:** Shallow anterior chamber as a sign of non-surgical choroidal detachment. Ann Ophthalmol 6:317, 1974
13. **Seelenfreund MH, Kraushar MF, Schepens CL, Freilich DB:** Choroidal detachment associated with primary retinal detachment. Arch Ophthalmol 91:254, 1974
14. **Tsukahara I, Uyama M:** Central serous retinopathy with bullous retinal detachment. Albrecht von Graefes Arch Klin Ophthalmol 206:169, 1978
15. **Yanoff M, Fine BS:** Ocular Pathology. Hagerstown, Harper & Row, 1975, pp 416–418

6

FUNDUS
EXAMINATION
AND
PREOPERATIVE
MANAGEMENT

INDIRECT OPHTHALMOSCOPY

PRINCIPLES AND ADVANTAGES

The first precept of retinal detachment surgery is that all the breaks must be found. The indirect ophthalmoscope is the best instrument for this purpose.[5, 7, 9, 10] In indirect ophthalmoscopy, a light source illuminates the patient's fundus; light rays diverging from this fundus are focused by a convex lens into an intermediate image, which is focused onto the examiner's fundus (Fig. 6-1). The image perceived by the latter is inverted and backward (Fig. 6-2).

The Schepens binocular indirect ophthalmoscope utilizes this basic system with certain additions which make it the best available indirect ophthalmoscope. The headpiece is constructed so that the light of a high–intensity electric lamp is focused onto a mirror which reflects the light onto the patient's fundus. Because the mirror is mounted above the view box, the beam of light entering the patient's eye (illumination beam) is separated from the light rays which are viewed by the examiner (observation beams). This arrangement prevents the corneal light reflex of the illumination beam from interfering with viewing (Fig. 6-3). The view box contains prisms which provide stereoscopic vision. They optically "narrow" the examiner's pupillary distance; otherwise, the light rays exiting from the patient's pupil could not reach both of the examiner's pupils (Fig. 6-4).

The indirect ophthalmoscope offers several advantages over the direct ophthalmoscope. First, the strong illumination provided by the head lamp plus the light gathering capability of the hand lens enable the examiner to see through hazy media. Second, it provides stereopsis. Third, indirect ophthalmoscopy, combined with scleral depression, provides the best view of the peripheral retina. Fourth, it makes a wide area of the retina visible at one time, thereby helping to insure that no abnormalities will be missed (Fig. 6-5).

TECHNIQUE

The large, aspheric lenses provide a sharper image and wider field of view than do the smaller, spheric lenses. As for power, the 14 diopter lens has the highest magnification (3.6 ×) of the commonly used lenses, but is difficult to use because of its long focal length (7 cm.). Examiners with small hands cannot steady the lens by resting their fingers on the patient's face. The 30 diopter lens (f = 3.3 cm.) is easy to use, but it gives inadequate magnification (1.5 ×)

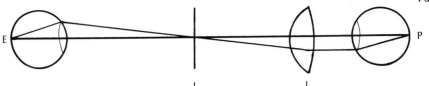

FIG. 6-1. Indirect ophthalmoscopy. (A) Rays from a point in the patient's fundus (P) are focused by a lens (L) into an intermediate image (I) which is viewed by the examiner (E).

FIG. 6-2. The relative position of rays of light a and b from points A and B in the patient's fundus is reversed at the intermediate image (I), so that a strikes the examiner's superior retina at A'. Since the examiner's inferior visual field is "seen" by his superior retina, A appears to be inferior to B.

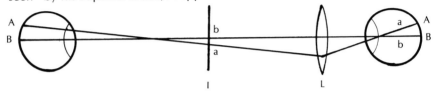

for finding small breaks. I prefer the 20 diopter lens (f=5 cm.), which is easy to use and provides a magnification of 2.3 ×.[10] Any lens should be held with the more convex surface toward the examiner (Fig. 6-1). It is slightly tilted to move the two light reflexes (one from each surface of the lens) away from the examiner's viewing axis (Fig. 6-6).

The patient should be reclining comfortably for the examination. The widest possible dilation of the pupil is desirable. Bilateral cycloplegia combined with topical anesthesia reduces photophobia and enhances cooperation. Bell's phenomenon is avoided if the patient keeps both eyes open. A fixation target such as the patient's thumb or a mark on the ceiling is helpful.

In order to minimize the corneal light reflex, the mirror must be adjusted so that the illumination beam is in the top of the field of view of the eye pieces. For small pupils, the light must be directed still higher (Fig. 6-7).

The superior periphery should be examined first because photophobia is minimized in upgaze and because the periphery is less sensitive to light than is the posterior pole. Initially, the transformer rheostat should be set at a low voltage. Higher light intensities can be used later, as the patient becomes less light-sensitive. Sensitivity to light is inversely proportional to the area of detached retina. A patient with a total retinal detachment will usually tolerate the full voltage.

Beginners frequently make the error of standing too close to the patient (Figs. 6-8, 6-9). It is much easier for the examiner to obtain a clear fundus image if his arm is extended. This is especially important if the pupil is small.

The examiner should hold his head so that he looks directly into the quadrant being examined. To examine the nasal periphery, he should stand on the same side as the eye being examined (Figs. 6-10, 6-11); for the temporal periphery, on the opposite side (Figs. 6-12, 6-13). The hand lens is shifted from

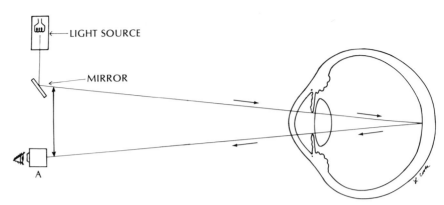

FIG. 6-3. The path of light rays entering the eye (illumination beam) is separated from those leaving it (observation beam), minimizing corneal light reflexes.

FIG. 6-4. Prisms in the view box of the binocular indirect ophthalmoscope "narrow" the examiner's pupillary distance. Therefore, from points in the patient's fundus, an observation beam (b) can reach each of the examiner's eyes. Without the viewbox, binocular vision would be impossible because light rays (a), aimed at each of the examiner's eyes, could not exit through the pupil.

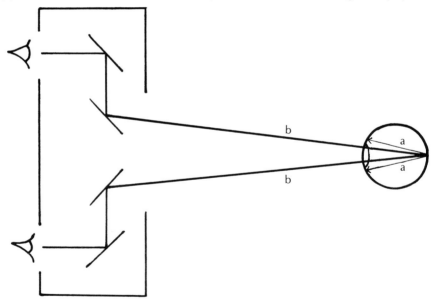

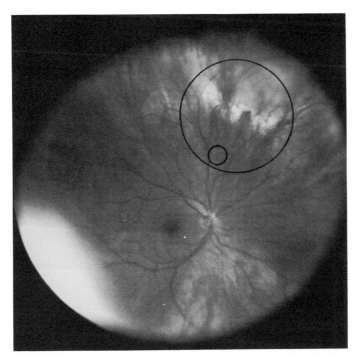

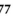

FIG. 6-5. The large circle indicates the area of the fundus which can be seen at one time with the indirect ophthalmoscope and the large 20 diopter lens. The small circle indicates the area which can be seen with the direct ophthalmoscope. Clearly, detection of the long-standing retinal detachment with demarcation line is easier with the indirect.

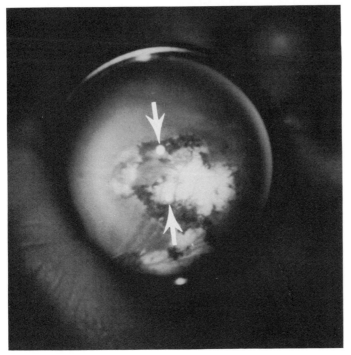

FIG. 6-6. Proper use of the hand lens. The lens is tilted to separate the light reflexes (*arrows*) on its surfaces.

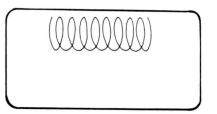 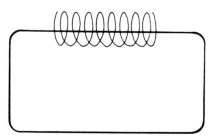

FIG. 6-7. For viewing through adequately dilated pupils (left), the reflected light (filament) should be at the top of the examiner's field of vision (*the enclosed area*). For viewing through small pupils (*right*), the mirror is positioned so that only a small strip of light is seen at the top of the field of vision.

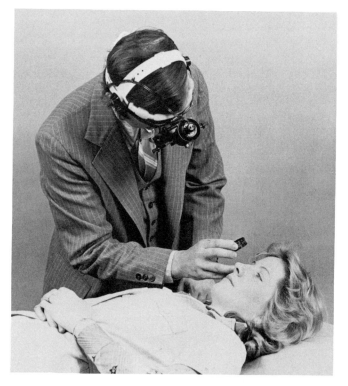

FIG. 6-8. Examiner standing too close to patient.

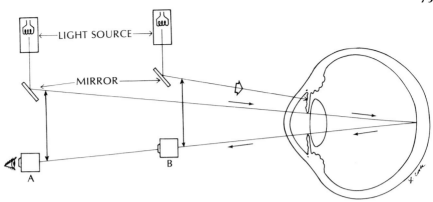

FIG. 6-9. The distance between the illumination beam and the observation beam(s) is fixed (*double-headed arrows*). When the examiner stands at position A, the illumination beam can enter the patient's pupil and the observation beam(s) can exit. At position B, the illumination beam (*open arrow*) cannot enter the eye. If the examiner lowered his head, the eye would be illuminated, but the observation beam(s) could not exit.

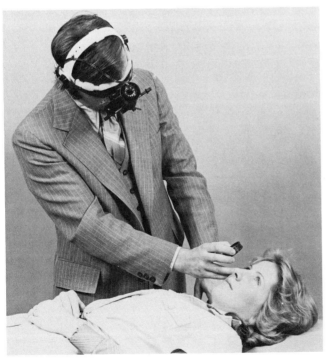

FIG. 6-10. Examination of the superonasal periphery, right eye. The patient keeps both eyes open and looks up and to the left. The examiner's arm is extended. He stands on the patient's right. He holds the lens in his right hand, steadying it by resting his finger on the patient's face.

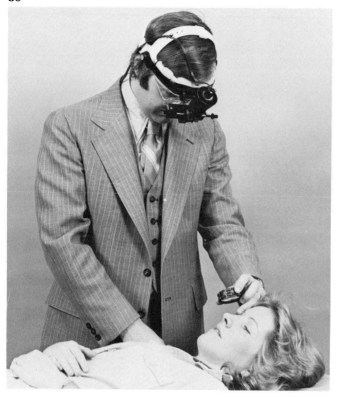

FIG. 6-11. Examination of inferonasal periphery, right eye. Patient looks down and left. The examiner remains on the patient's right but holds the lens in left hand.

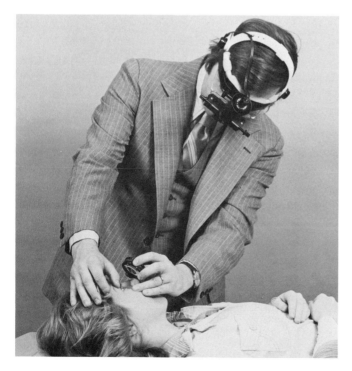

FIG. 6-12. Examination of superotemporal periphery, right eye. The examiner has moved to patient's left side. The lens is held in his left hand. The patient looks up and right. Her face is rolled to the left so that the nose is not an obstacle.

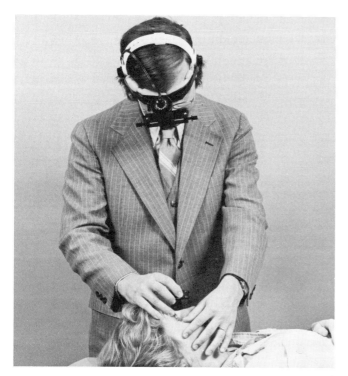

FIG. 6-13. Examination of the inferotemporal periphery, right eye. The examiner remains on the patient's left but has shifted the lens to his right hand.

FIG. 6-14. (*A*) Examiner's head is incorrectly positioned for examination of the temporal periphery. (*B*) Examiner's head is properly tilted so that the eye is well illuminated and a monocular image can be seen.

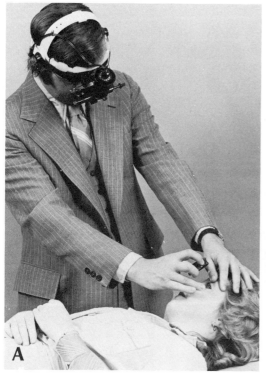

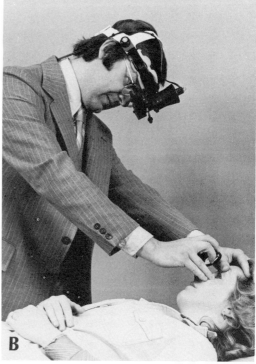

his right to left hand as necessary to avoid awkward maneuvering, especially during scleral depression. The nose becomes less of an obstacle to viewing the temporal periphery when the patient rolls his head toward the examiner while looking temporally.

The pupillary aperture appears elliptical to the examiner when he looks at the peripheral retina. This makes stereoscopic viewing more difficult and decreases the amount of light which can enter the eye. The examiner must increase the voltage of his light source and tilt his head slightly so that part of the illumination beam can enter the eye and one of the observation beams can exit (Figs, 6-14, 6-15). This achieves only a monocular view.

THE FUNDUS DRAWING

A detailed drawing of the fundus should be made prior to surgery. The drawing may help locate the tears during surgery if the media become opaque or if the pupil constricts. Retinal hemorrhages, pigment, blood vessels, and folds should be represented. On the standard diagrams commonly used, the outermost circle represents the pars plicata of the ciliary body; the second, the ora serrata; and the innermost, the equator, which is located two disc diameters anterior to the ampullae of the vortex veins (Fig. 6-16).

There are two ways to correct for the inverted image of the indirect ophthalmoscope. The first is to observe the retina, then mentally correct for the inverted image, drawing the findings as they are, not as they are seen. The second method is to invert the drawing pad and then to draw the findings as they are seen. When the drawing is finished, the findings will be correctly positioned.

After the limits of the detachment have been sketched, all retinal breaks must be found. To this end, one may start at the optic nerve and follow each of the retinal vessels to the periphery. A scanning technique should also be used. Keeping his eyes and the hand lens aligned, the examiner swings his gaze along the periphery (Fig. 6-17). This serves two purposes. First, the entire retina is examined. Second, holes can be recognized when a sudden change in the brightness of the subretinal layers is noted. A hole is perceived as a discontinuity in the nearly uniform translucency of the detached retina (Fig. 6-18); when the observer's gaze is moving, the discontinuity becomes easier to see because of the contrast between the detached retina and the now visible layers underneath (Fig. 6-19). Slightly wiggling the lens from side to side produces a prism effect which also helps to reveal discontinuities in the retina (Fig. 6-20).

SCLERAL DEPRESSION

After the retina has been thoroughly scanned, the peripheral retina should be examined with scleral depression to detect small holes, especially those near the ora serrata. In some patients, this region cannot be seen at all without indentation. Beginners should not attempt scleral depression until they are adept at viewing the retina anterior to the equator with the indirect ophthalmoscope. Otherwise, the scleral depression will afford little or no information and the patient will have suffered needlessly.

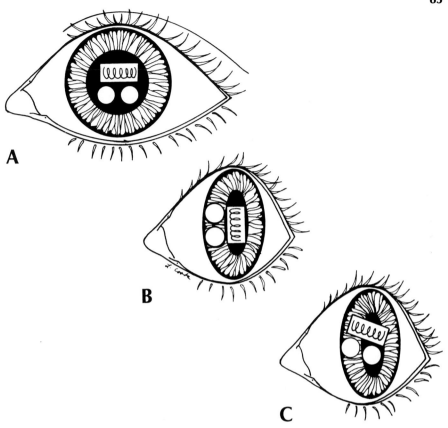

FIG. 6-15. (*A*) Viewing the posterior pole through a large pupil. The illumination beam (filament) enters through the top leaving ample room for the observation beams (*white circles*) below. Binocular vision is provided. (*B*) The pupillary aperture becomes elliptical when the examiner tries to see the far periphery. If he does not tilt his head, the illumination beam can enter the eye, but the observation beams cannot emerge. (*C*) The examiner must tilt his head so that part of the illumination beam can enter the eye. Often only a monocular view of the fundus is possible, as only one of the observation beams can emerge from the eye.

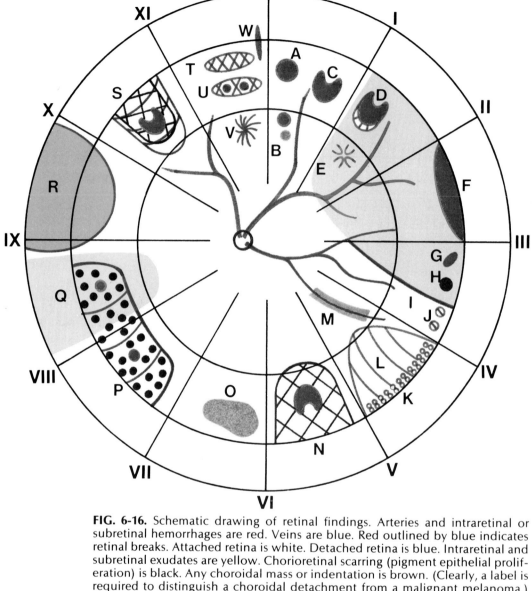

FIG. 6-16. Schematic drawing of retinal findings. Arteries and intraretinal or subretinal hemorrhages are red. Veins are blue. Red outlined by blue indicates retinal breaks. Attached retina is white. Detached retina is blue. Intraretinal and subretinal exudates are yellow. Chorioretinal scarring (pigment epithelial proliferation) is black. Any choroidal mass or indentation is brown. (Clearly, a label is required to distinguish a choroidal detachment from a malignant melanoma.) Anything in the vitreous (hemorrhage, foreign body, etc.) is green. Here, too, a label is often required. (A) round hole; (B) operculated tear; (C) flap tear; (D) flap tear with posteriorly rolled edge; (E) fixed fold; (F) retinal dialysis (disinsertion); (G) retinal hemorrhage; (H) intraretinal pigmentation; (I) demarcation line; (J) cobblestones; (K) peripheral cystoid degeneration; (L) senile retinoschisis; (M) exudate along a retinal artery; (N) flap tear surrounded by cryotherapy scarring; (O) vitreous opacity (needs label); (P) two round holes on a circumferential scleral buckle surrounded by diathermy scars. Superiorly, the retina has redetached; (Q) detachment of non-pigmented epithelium of the pars plana; (R) choroidal mass (needs label); (S) flap tear surrounded by cryotherapy scarring on a radial scleral buckle; (T) lattice degeneration; (U) lattice degeneration with atrophic round holes; (V) vortex vein ampulla; (W) meridional fold. (See color plate.)

I prefer the original thimble-type depressor designed by Schepens, although a simple cotton-tipped applicator can also be used.

Scleral depression helps in three ways to detect small breaks. First, it increases the contrast between the intact retina and the break. The indented choroid/retinal pigment epithelium is darker than the unindented choiroid/retinal pigment epithelium and darker still than the intact retina, enabling the examiner to locate the break, which appears as a dark spot (Figs. 6-21, 6-22). Second, the decreased retinal translucency which results from scleral depression may increase the contrast between the hole and the retina, allowing the hole to be seen. The retina appears less translucent because it is seen at a more acute angle (Fig. 6-23). Moreover, the increased angle may aid the examiner to see the posterior edge of a break. Third, the flaps of tiny breaks at the posterior vitreous base can sometimes be seen as the sclera is indented (Fig. 6-24). In all cases, constant movement of the scleral depressor maximizes the chances of finding a small break.

Scleral depression does not enlarge retinal holes and there are very few contraindications to its use. It should be avoided only in patients who have had recent intraocular surgery. Scleral depression may cause pain. It raises the intraocular pressure and is therefore especially painful in eyes with a high initial pressure. Glaucoma patients must be examined very gently. Also, the examination stretches and compresses the eyelids and may thereby cause discomfort. To minimize this, scleral depression should be started superiorly because the upper lid is looser and more flexible than the lower.

The patient looks down and the examiner places the depressor near the lid margin, following the eyelid up as the patient looks up. Beginners should hold the depressor vertically so that the indentation can be found easily with the indirect ophthalmoscope. The examiner merely follows the shaft of the depressor down into the eye. If he does not see the indentation, he should scan the fundus, moving his head from side to side. Vertical depression also simplifies the problem of orienting one's movements in the inverted upside-down field of the indirect ophthalmoscope (Fig. 6-25). Anterior-posterior movements are easily made. If the observer wants to examine further posteriorly, he simply moves the depressor toward the optic nerve. Circumferential movements are more difficult, but they become automatic with practice. The beginner simply has to remember that the depressor should be moved opposite to the direction suggested by his view of the retina.

If the ora serrata is to be viewed, the patient should look as far superiorly as possible (Fig. 6-26). Beginners will see the ora serrata most easily in highly myopic eyes and in aphakic eyes which have had a sector iridectomy. If areas of the superior retina posterior to the equator are to be examined, the patient must look slightly inferiorly (Fig. 6-27).

Scleral depression is most difficult at the 9:00 and 3:00 positions because the eyelid is shorter here and because the canthal ligaments resist the posterior movement of the depressor. Direct scleral depression at the canthus is painful. Moreover, the depressor may slip off the eyelid and strike the patient's eye. The following techniques help to avoid these problems. First, the depressor is placed on the superior eyelid, above the horizontal axis. It is then rotated downward toward the canthus, carrying the eyelid down with it. The lid be-

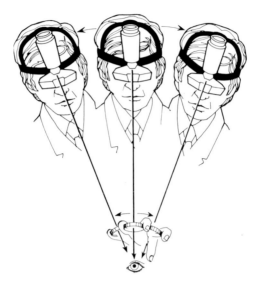

FIG. 6-17. Scanning technique for examining the retina. The examiner keeps his eyes and lens aligned while viewing the retina.

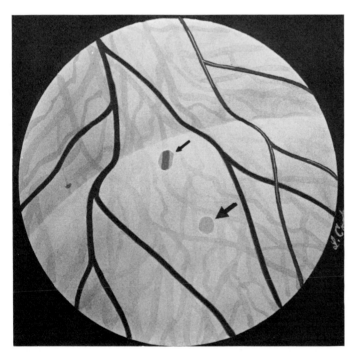

FIG. 6-18. Retinal breaks are perceived as discontinuities in the detached retina. One hole (*small arrow*) appears as a dark spot because a choroidal vessel underlies it. The other (*large arrow*) is more difficult to see because of lack of contrast between the retina and the subretinal layers.

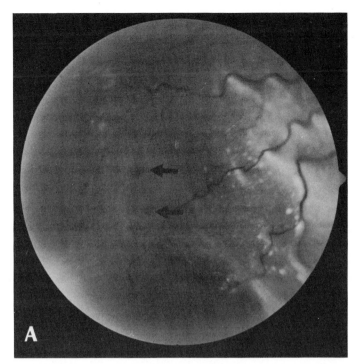

FIG. 6-19. Retinal detachment with two small holes (*arrows*) in a patch of lattice degeneration. Under the detachment is an area of nonpigmented choroid. (*A*) The superior hole appears to be a dark spot. The inferior hole appears as a light spot.

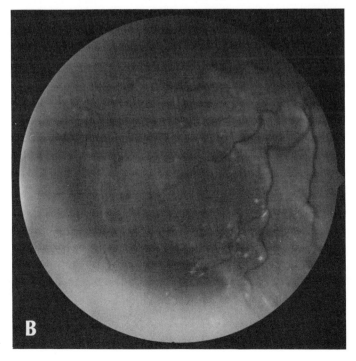

(*B*) Viewed from a different angle, the superior hole appears to be a light spot. The inferior hole appears to be a dark spot.

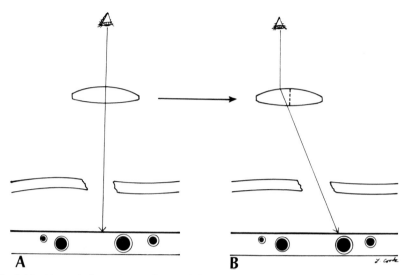

FIG. 6-20. Use of the prism effect of the lens to find retinal breaks. (*A*) Break initially difficult to find because of little contrast between the detached retina and the background. (*B*) As lens moves, the retina appears to move with it. A choroidal vessel is suddenly seen more clearly, identifying the break.

FIG. 6-21. Scleral depression changes the brightness of the subretinal layers. (*A*) Without indentation light rays 3, 4, and 5 are reflected directly back to the examiner. (*B*) With indentation, some light rays are reflected away from the examiner, so that the indented area appears darker.

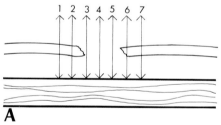

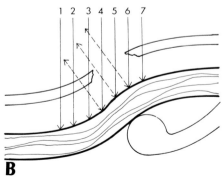

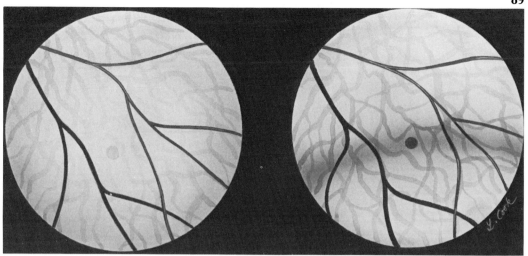

FIG. 6-22. The use of scleral depression to find retinal breaks. Left, the retinal hole can barely be seen because of little contrast between the retina and the underlying choroid. Right, scleral depression darkens the underlying choroid. The hole is seen as a dark spot.

FIG. 6-23. (*A*) Without scleral depression, light rays have a short path through the retina. (*B*) Retina tilted by scleral depression. The light rays must travel a longer path through the retina, which therefore appears less translucent.

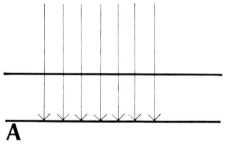

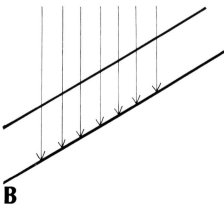

comes more slack when the patient, his head rolled away from the examiner, is not looking into an extreme position of gaze (Fig. 6-28).[3] Second, a cotton-tipped applicator, being blunter and softer than a metal depressor, may be better tolerated. Finally, if the above techniques have been unsuccessful, one can easily depress directly on the conjunctiva after topical anesthesia has been administered (Fig. 6-29).

After thoroughly examining the retina with indirect ophthalmoscopy and scleral depression, one should use the slit lamp and the Goldmann three-mirror lens to search for small breaks and to evaluate vitreous traction. It is essential that the fellow eye be carefully examined for retinal breaks or other abnormalities which might require prophylactic treatment.[2]

FINDING THE RETINAL BREAKS

The configuration of the retinal detachment suggests the location of at least one retinal break.[8] The basic principle is that gravity helps subretinal fluid to dissect inferiorly and retards superior dissection. The following hints may be helpful:

1. For superior retinal detachments crossing the 12:00 meridian, a break will be within 1½ hours of 12:00 on the side with the greatest inferior extent of detachment (Fig. 6-30).

2. For retinal detachments involving the superior retina but not crossing the 12:00 meridian, a break will be within 1½ hours of the most superior edge of the detachment (Fig. 6-31).

3. A focal spot of pigment may help to locate a break because such a spot sometimes appears in the flap of a tiny horseshoe tear (Fig. 6-31).

4. For inferior detachments higher on one side, a break will be located on that side (Fig. 6-32).

5. For inferior detachments with equal upward extent on both sides, a break will usually be found near 6:00 (Fig. 6-33).

6. Inferior breaks usually do not cause highly bullous retinal detachments. Therefore, when large bullae are seen inferiorly, the surgeon must look carefully for a superior retinal break.

7. When no breaks are found in an inferior retinal detachment, a superior break may be leaking fluid down a shallow peripheral trough (Fig. 6-34). Locating these breaks is sometimes facilitated by having the patient's head tilted far backwards, allowing the fluid to shift up toward the break (Fig. 6-35).

8. If a demarcation line is present, there must be a hole between the line and the ora serrata (Fig. 6-36).

9. Until proven otherwise, one should suspect that a break is present at the end of meridional folds, especially in aphakic retinal detachments.

10. In aphakic retinal detachments, the surgeon should carefully examine the posterior border of the vitreous base for tiny flap tears (Fig. 6-24).[1]

11. In high myopes with a posterior staphyloma, a break may be found anywhere in the posterior pole, not necessarily in the fovea.

12. In redetachments, the surgeon should first see if the original break or breaks have reopened (Fig. 6-37). If not, a break may be found in the most superior area where subretinal fluid crosses over the scleral buckle (Fig. 6-38).

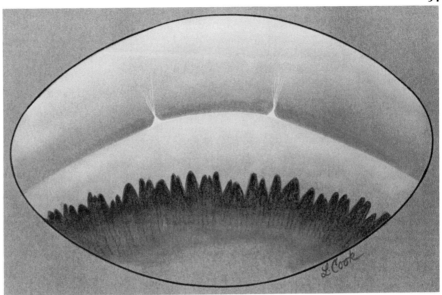

FIG. 6-24. Indirect ophthalmoscopic view of tiny flap tears with vitreous traction, demonstrated by scleral depression at the posterior vitreous base.

FIG. 6-25. (*A*) Incorrect technique for scleral depression. It is difficult to make diagonal correcting movements because of the upside down and backward image of the indirect ophthalmoscope. (*B*) Correct technique for scleral depression. The depressor is held vertically so that horizontal and vertical correcting movements can be easily made.

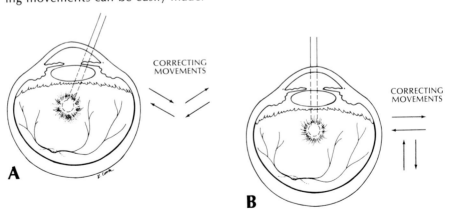

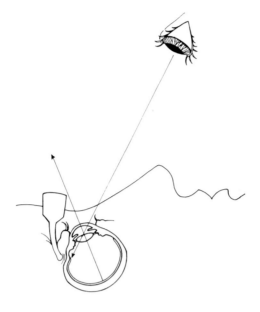

FIG. 6-26. The ora serrata can be seen best when the patient looks as far superiorly as possible.

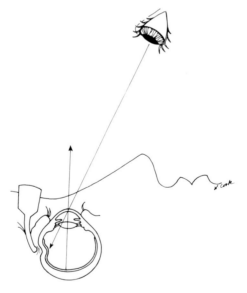

FIG. 6-27. In order to view the midperiphery, the examiner should have the patient look slightly inferiorly.

FIG. 6-29. Examination of the temporal periphery. If the eyelid is not slack ▶ enough to allow depression, the scleral depressor can be placed on the anesthetized conjunctiva.

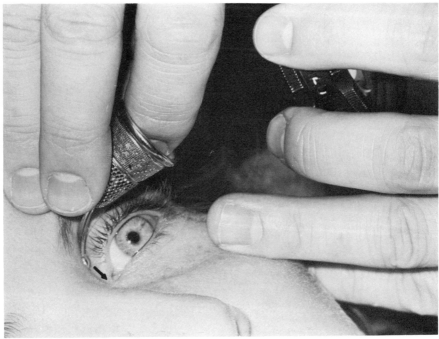

FIG. 6-28. Scleral depression of the nasal periphery. The patient's head is rolled away from the examiner. She looks straight ahead, keeping the lid slack. The scleral depressor is placed on the superior eyelid above the horizontal axis. It is then rotated downward toward the canthus (*arrow*), carrying the eyelid with it.

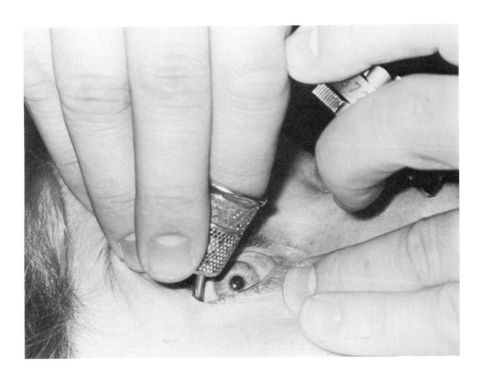

If no subretinal fluid crosses over the buckle, the break is probably posterior to it (Fig. 6-39).

13. When a break is not easily located, the patient should be examined in a sitting position. The slight shift of the fluid may facilitate the detection of breaks.

14. In 3 to 10 per cent of patients with retinal detachment, no definite break is ever found.[4]

15. When a bullous retinal detachment is present, a break previously hidden by retinal folds sometimes appears after the subretinal fluid has been drained at surgery.

The above discussion in no way implies that the remainder of the retina need not be examined after a break has been found in the expected location. Fifty per cent of retinal detachments have more than one break.[9] If any retinal break is not closed, the surgery will fail.

PREOPERATIVE MANAGEMENT

MEDICAL EVALUATION

A careful medical evaluation is important, especially if the retinal detachment procedure, which often lasts 2 or more hours, is to be done under general anesthesia. Allergies must be identified. The anesthesiologist must be alerted if the patient has glaucoma and is being treated with anticholinesterase drugs, such as phospholine iodine. Because these drugs lower blood pseudocholinesterase, succinylcholine should not be used in conjunction with general anesthesia, or the patient will have prolonged respiratory paralysis.

PREVENTION OF INFECTION

Blepharoconjunctivitis, when present, should be treated before retinal surgery. Even in the absence of clinical infection, some surgeons routinely treat patients preoperatively with prophylactic antibiotics. The eyelashes are trimmed so that they do not contaminate the operative field and so that postoperative secretions can be more readily wiped away.

BINOCULAR PATCHING

Binocular patching and bed rest will, in almost all cases, prevent the spread of the retinal detachment. Moreover, significant quantities of subretinal fluid may be absorbed, especially in recent retinal detachments with small retinal breaks. The fluid is not as readily absorbed in aphakic and inferior retinal detachments.[7] The decreased elevation of the detachment facilitates the localization of breaks and sometimes allows a non-drainage procedure to be performed.

PUPILLARY DILATATION

After a complete eye examination, the patient receives scopolamine ¼ per

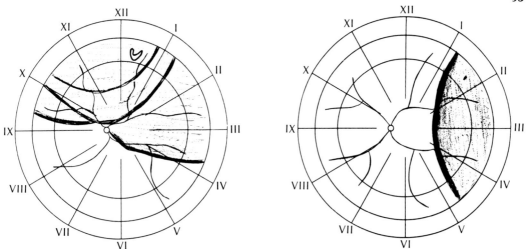

FIG. 6-30. Top, left. A superior retinal detachment which crosses the 12:00 meridian. A break is found near 12:00 on the side with the greatest inferior extent of detachment, in this case the temporal side.

FIG. 6-31. Top, right. A superior retinal detachment which does not cross the 12:00 meridian. A break is found within 1½ hours of its most superior margin. A focal pigmented spot alerts the examiner to the location of the break, which can only be seen with scleral depression.

FIG. 6-32. Bottom, left. An inferior detachment which is higher on the nasal side. A break is located on that side (at 8:45).

FIG. 6-33. Bottom, right. An inferior detachment with equal superior extent on both sides. A break is found near 6:00.

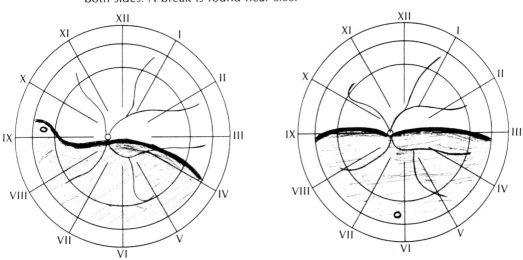

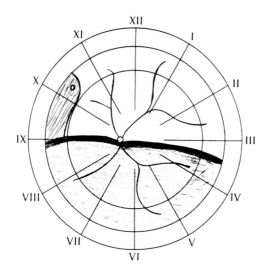

FIG. 6-34. When no inferior break is found in an inferior retinal detachment, the examiner should look for a superior break which is leaking fluid along a shallow peripheral trough.

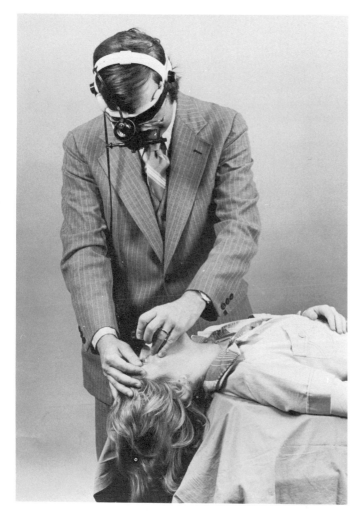

FIG. 6-35. Patient's neck is hyperextended to allow fluid to shift superiorly.

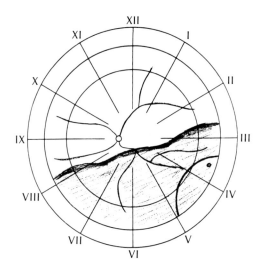

FIG. 6-36. A demarcation line (from 3:30 to 5:00) has failed to contain a retinal detachment. A break must be present between the demarcation line and the ora serrata.

FIG. 6-37. Redetached retina. (*A*) The encircling scleral buckle (*parallel curved lines*) was not placed far enough posteriorly to seal the horseshoe tear. (*B*) The segmental circumferential buckle was not placed far enough anteriorly.

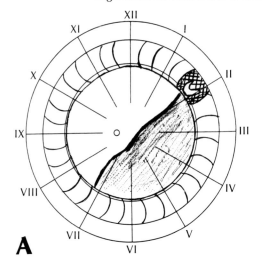

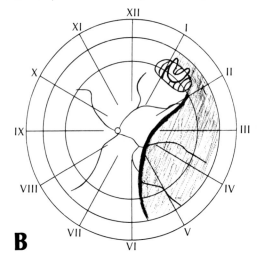

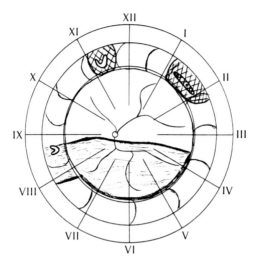

FIG. 6-38. Redetached retina. A break is often found where the subretinal fluid crosses over the scleral buckle (8:00 to 9:00).

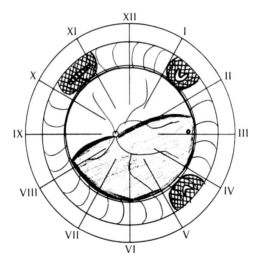

FIG. 6-39. Redetached retina. No fluid crosses over the scleral buckle. A break is found posterior to the buckle (3:00).

cent in both eyes twice per day. This avoids the need for repeated dilatation each time another member of the operating team examines the patient. Maximal cycloplegia and mydriasis are obtained if, beginning 1 hour before surgery, three applications of cyclopentolate 1 per cent and phenylephrine 10 per cent are given at 15-minute intervals. If the pupil will not dilate enough to allow peripheral retinal examination, it must be enlarged either by photocoagulation of the iris or by iridectomy. Iridectomy is also indicated in patients with angle closure glaucoma. If a dense cataract prevents satisfactory examination, it must be removed. Current techniques of cataract wound closure allow the cataract extraction and retinal surgery to be performed at one sitting.

REFERENCES

1. **Ashrafzadeh MT, Schepens CL, Elzeneiny IH, Moura R, Morse P, Kraushar M:** Aphakic and phakic retinal detachment. Arch Ophthalmol 89:476, 1973
2. **Benson WE:** Prophylactic therapy of retinal breaks. Surv Ophthalmol 22:41, 1977
3. **Curtin VT:** Management of retinal detachment. In Duane TD (ed): Clinical Ophthalmology, Vol 5, Surgery. Hagerstown, Harper & Row, 1978, p 2
4. **Griffith RD, Ryan EA, Hilton GF:** Primary retinal detachments without apparent breaks. Am J Ophthalmol 81:420, 1976
5. **Havener WH, Gloeckner S:** Atlas of Diagnostic Techniques and Treatment of Retinal Detachment. St. Louis, CV Mosby, 1967, pp 2–53
6. **Hofmann H, Hanselmayer H:** Frequency and extent of spontaneous flattening of retinal detachments by patient immobilization. Klin Monatsbl Augenheilkd 162:178, 1973
7. **Hovland KR, Elzeneiny IH, Schepens CL:** Clinical evaluation of the small pupil binocular indirect ophthalmoscope. Arch Ophthalmol 82:466, 1969
8. **Lincoff H, Gieser R:** Finding the retinal hole. Arch Ophthalmol 85:565, 1971
9. **Rosenthal ML, Fradin S:** The technique of binocular indirect ophthalmoscopy. Highlights of Ophthalmology 9:179–257, 1967
10. **Rubin ML:** The optics of indirect ophthalmoscopy. Surv Ophthalmol 9:449, 1964

7

BASIC
SURGICAL
TECHNIQUE

ANESTHESIA

Retrobulbar anesthesia has three advantages over general anesthesia: Total operating-room time is decreased, there is less bleeding, and operative mortality may be slightly decreased.[15] Its possible complications are perforation of the globe,[32] retrobulbar hemorrhage, central retinal artery occlusion,[19] and more difficult exposure during surgery. In addition, the patient may experience pain during the procedure, may become disoriented and restless if he is oversedated, or may have discomfort from having to lie still during a long procedure. One cannot always predict that an operation will be "easy" or short. Occasionally, unexpected findings or operative complications necessitate a longer procedure than originally planned. Because we feel that the disadvantages of local anesthesia outweigh its advantages, we use general anesthesia for retinal detachment surgery at the Wills Eye Hospital.

OPENING

In initial operations, the peritomy can be made either at the limbus or 4 mm. from it. The limbal peritomy[18] has several advantages: It is opened and closed faster, requires less suture material for closure, covers the site of surgery with an intact layer of tissue, causes less bleeding, does not shorten the fornices, is less likely to cause symblepharon, and causes less postoperative adhesion of Tenon's capsule to the sclera, thereby facilitating reoperation. The limbal conjunctiva and Tenon's capsule are tented up with toothed forceps and are incised down to the sclera with blunt scissors (Fig. 7-1). Tenon's capsule is separated from the perilimbal sclera by blunt dissection so that a 360° incision can be made as close to the limbus as possible (Fig. 7-2). (When a single radial sponge [see below] is to be placed, a 180° incision suffices.) Two relaxing incisions (Fig. 7-3), 180° apart, serve to avoid tearing the conjunctiva. Additional blunt dissection between Tenon's capsule and the sclera is performed posteriorly (Fig. 7-4) so that the rectus muscles can be hooked and bridled. A 4-0 black silk suture is passed under the muscle and tied. Before proceeding further, the surgeon must look for areas of thin sclera. Otherwise, he may perforate the globe during localization. In the rare cases in which adequate exposure cannot be obtained, a lateral canthotomy is performed, and one or more muscles are disinserted. A traction suture is placed into the stump of the tendon.

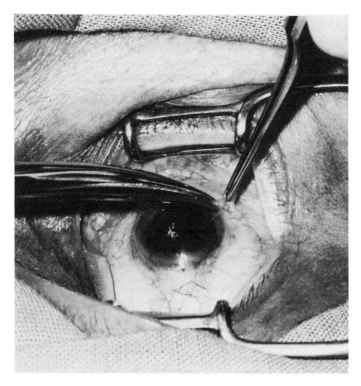

FIG. 7-1. Limbal peritomy. The conjunctiva and Tenon's capsule are tented up with toothed forceps and incised with blunt scissors.

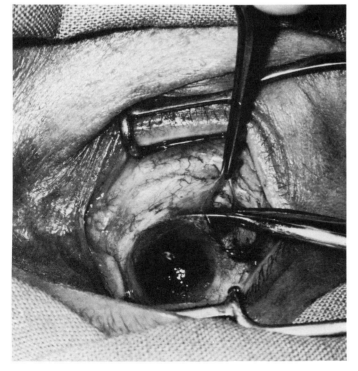

FIG. 7-2. Tenon's capsule is undermined by blunt dissection so that the incision can be as close to the limbus as possible.

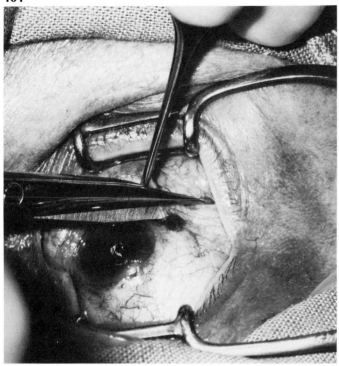

FIG. 7-3. Radial relaxing incision.

FIG. 7-4. (*A*) Posteriorly, Tenon's capsule is loosely adherent to the sclera. (*B*) Blunt dissection easily separates Tenon's capsule from the sclera.

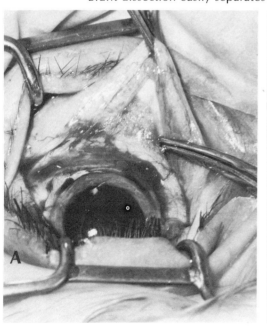

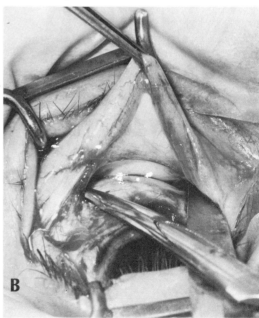

LOCALIZATION

In order to correctly place the scleral buckle, the surgeon must localize all breaks which the buckle is to cover (i.e., the sclera underlying them must be marked). I localize with a blunt-tipped diathermy electrode, using the indirect ophthalmoscope for visualization. The intensity of the diathermy should first be tested on anterior sclera to insure an adequate but not excessive scleral coagulation. Then the assistant steadies the eye by holding two bridle sutures while the surgeon, using a cotton-tipped applicator for scleral depression, locates the meridian of the break. The diathermy electrode is next introduced into this meridian. Keeping his wrist cocked to ensure that only the tip of the instrument indents the sclera, the surgeon makes a few gentle applications of diathermy on the sclera underlying the retinal break. The eye is then rolled forward and additional diathermy is applied to make a permanent mark (Fig. 7-5).

For small breaks, the posterior edge alone is localized; for large flap tears, the posterior edge and both anterior horns; for lattice degeneration with holes, both ends of the degeneration; for dialyses, the ends of the dialysis as well as the point in the center of the dialysis where the surgeon estimates that the retina will fall. Anterior and posterior localization of long tears is very important, since many are not radial in direction (Fig. 7-6).

If either a staphyloma or very thin sclera is present in the region of the hole, the diathermy technique is dangerous because the electrode may penetrate the globe. A less sharp instrument, such as the wooden end of a cotton-tipped applicator, is used to indent and temporarily mark the sclera underlying the tear. The eye is then rolled forward and gentle applications of diathermy make a permanent mark.

In highly bullous detachments, parallax can lead the surgeon to localize more posteriorly than the actual position of the break (Fig. 7-7). He can minimize the error by first localizing the least elevated part of the break, generally its anterior border. This then serves as a reference point as he gently slides the electrode posteriorly under indirect ophthalmoscopic control until he judges that the posterior border of the break has been reached (Fig. 7-8). In rare cases, accurate localization of the breaks can be achieved only after the retina has been flattened by a combination of drainage of the subretinal fluid and an injection of saline into the vitreous cavity.

Finally, after the known breaks have been localized, the surgeon must fully reinspect the retina for any which may have been missed. If the preoperative examination has been difficult, this final check is all the more important.

TREATMENT MODALITIES

A firm adhesion between the retina and either the retinal pigment epithelium or the choroid is required to adequately seal retinal breaks. Diathermy and cryotherapy are the modalities most frequently used to induce this adhesion.

DIATHERMY

Unlike other forms of electricity, diathermy (radiofrequency electric current) is not conducted by body tissues to distant sites such as the heart. When it is

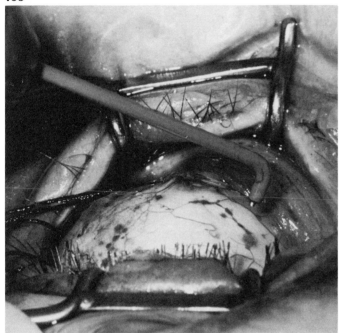

FIG. 7-5. The diathermy coagulation is reinforced to make a permanent mark.

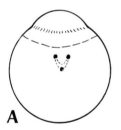

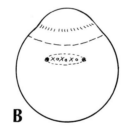

A

B

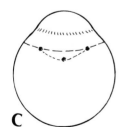

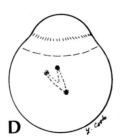

C

D

FIG. 7-6. Localization technique for flap tears (*A*), lattice degeneration (*B*), retinal dialyses (*C*), and long tears (*D*). The broken line represents the ora serrata.

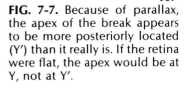

FIG. 7-7. Because of parallax, the apex of the break appears to be more posteriorly located (Y') than it really is. If the retina were flat, the apex would be at Y, not at Y'.

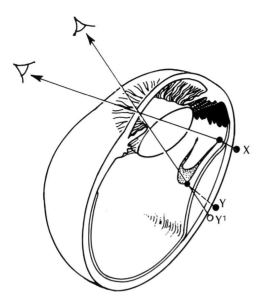

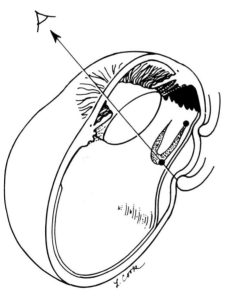

FIG. 7-8. Errors induced by parallax can be minimized if the less elevated anterior horn is localized first. Then the localizing instrument, functioning as a scleral depressor, is slid posteriorly under indirect ophthalmoscopic control until the surgeon determines that the apex has been reached. He then marks the sclera at this point.

applied to the sclera, a focal coagulation of the sclera, choroid, and pigment epithelium results. Applications are made 2 mm. apart in the bed of a lamellar scleral dissection (see below). When the retina is brought into contact with the treated areas, a chorioretinal scar develops.

CRYOTHERAPY

Freezing focally destroys the choriocapillaris, retinal pigment epithelium, and outer retinal layers. A firm chorioretinal scar is the result. Some experienced retinal surgeons feel that an adequate adhesion results from cryotherapy of the pigment epithelium surrounding a break, even if the overlying detached retina is not frozen.[13] Experimental evidence indicates, however, that such treatment results in a relationship between the sensory retina and the pigment epithelium similar to the relatively weak adhesion found in eyes without detachment.[20] A histologically strong adhesion results when the pigment epithelium and the sensory retina are both frozen during treatment, for tight junctions are later seen between Müller cells and the pigment epithelium. Freezing the pigment epithelium within the break does not increase the strength of the adhesion. Such freezing only releases more pigment into the vitreous and the subretinal fluid.

The pressure of the cryoprobe on the sclera forces fluid from the eye. As the eye softens, high indentation by the probe is possible. Therefore, breaks in attached retina should be frozen first; breaks in highly detached retina, last. As the assistant steadies the eye with the rectus muscle bridle sutures, the surgeon, viewing with the indirect ophthalmoscope, surrounds the tears with 2 to 3 mm. of retinal freezing to insure adequate adhesion. It is important that he keep his wrist cocked outward so that only the tip of the cryoprobe indents the eye. Beginners tend to indent the eye with the shaft of the probe, mistaking this indentation for the indentation of the probe's tip. When treatment is then applied, the freezing tip of the probe can cause severe damage beyond the area of visualization. Most cryoprobes have a small knob 180° away from the freezing tip to aid the surgeon in orienting the probe. The freezing portion of the tip must be pressed squarely against the globe. After the first application, the surgeon keeps the probe in place until the iceball has thawed; then, watching retinal landmarks, he gently slides the probe sufficiently to place the next contiguous lesion. An alternative method of treatment allows the surgeon to check the accuracy of his localization marks. Under direct visualization, he freezes the probe to the mark. He then rolls the eye backward to verify his treatment with the indirect ophthalmoscope. Retinal freezing is observed surrounding the break if the localization mark is correct (Fig. 7-9).

The firmer the indentation, the faster the rate of freezing because choroidal blood flow (an insulator) is stopped. Excessive indentation can close the central retinal artery. After a few consecutive applications, the surgeon must relax the pressure on the eye to permit ocular circulation. If a break is highly elevated, the surgeon should not indent excessively, especially if the patient has recently undergone intraocular surgery or if he has staphylomatous sclera. When these conditions are present, the subretinal fluid should be drained prior to cryotherapy.

The sensory retina becomes slightly less transparent when frozen; this opacification helps the surgeon to verify that his treatment applications have been contiguous. Scleral depression makes this change easier to see. The opaqueness also aids in differentiating small retinal breaks from small patches of thin retina. Normal and thin retina both turn white when frozen. Full-thickness retinal breaks appear dark in contrast to the adjacent frozen retina.

CRYOTHERAPY VERSUS DIATHERMY

There is some controversy over whether diathermy or cryotherapy should be used in retinal detachment surgery.[13, 26, 34] Both of these techniques yield good results, though each has its advantages and disadvantages.

Advantages of Cryotherapy over Diathermy

Unlike diathermy, cryotherapy causes little or no scleral damage[35] and provides adequate treatment through full-thickness sclera, obviating scleral dissection and allowing the use of explants for scleral buckling. Infections following a procedure in which cryotherapy has been used are less likely to cause endophthalmitis than are infections following scleral dissection and diathermy.[25] In addition, since the sclera has not been disturbed, reoperations are performed easily and safely.

Unlike diathermy, which cannot be applied over the long ciliary arteries or vortex veins without occluding them, cryotherapy causes no damage to either.[10] Cryotherapy can be applied safely over staphylomatous sclera without further damaging it, provided care is taken to allow the ice ball to thaw completely before the probe is removed. Cryotherapy safely treats the retina, whereas diathermy can cause a retinal hole. Cryotherapy forces fluid from the eye and may allow adequate indentation of the scleral buckle without drainage of the subretinal fluid. Because it shrinks the sclera, diathermy raises the intraocular pressure and thereby generally necessitates the drainage of subretinal fluid. Only cryotherapy is effective on wet sclera, e.g., after premature release of subretinal fluid.

Advantages of Diathermy over Cryotherapy

Since cryotherapy lesions must be contiguous to seal retinal holes, great care must be taken not to miss any part of the border of the tear. Diathermy lesions, on the other hand, need not be contiguous. Therefore, even treatment is applied quickly and large areas of normal pigment epithelium and choroid remain undisturbed. For this reason, it may be easier to find small holes in redetached retina after diathermy than after cryotherapy.[34] Cryotherapy also disrupts retinal pigment epithelial cells, causing pigment fallout under the retina. Diathermy does not. This probably does not cause visual loss,[14] but the resultant depigmentation of the pigment epithelium eliminates the color contrast which might help the examiner to locate small holes in thinned redetached retina.

In highly myopic and senile eyes, especially if the sclera is too vigorously indented, cryotherapy may break Bruch's membrane and cause a subretinal hemorrhage. There is no firm clinical evidence that either treatment modality

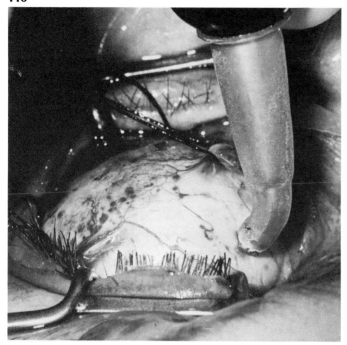

FIG. 7-9. Checking the accuracy of localization. The cryoprobe tip is frozen to the localization mark. The eye is then rolled backward for indirect ophthalmoscopy. The surgeon should be able to confirm proper placement of the treatment by observing freezing of the retina surrounding the break.

FIG. 7-10. (*A*) Principle of scleral buckling. Retinal detachment caused by flap tear due to vitreous traction. (*B*) Vitreous traction sufficiently relieved by indentation of a radial sponge. Detachment cured.

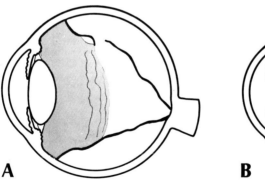
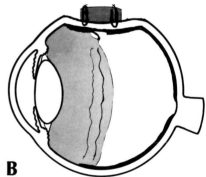

A   B

results in a stronger final adhesion. Some surgeons believe, however, that a "sticky exudate" makes the early adhesion of diathermy firmer.[34]

SCLERAL BUCKLING PROCEDURES

Indenting the sclera and choroid toward the retinal breaks ("scleral buckling") facilitates settling of the detached retina and may make a non-drainage procedure possible. In addition, scleral buckling relieves vitreous traction (Fig. 7-10), which, if unrelieved, can reopen a retinal break despite cryotherapy or diathermy treatment. Either an implant or an explant serves to buckle the sclera.

EXPLANTS

An explant is a foreign material attached by sutures to the sclera. Explants may be radial (perpendicular to the ora serrata) or circumferential (parallel to the ora serrata). The latter may be encircling or segmental. All explant material currently used is made of silicone. There are two varieties: silicone sponge and solid silicone. Available sponges are 80 mm. long and are either round (3, 4, and 5 mm. in diameter) or elliptical (7.5 × 5.5 mm.). Solid silicone is available in a variety of sizes and shapes. Explants are held in place by mattress sutures of 5-0 monofilament nylon, 4-0 or 5-0 dacron, or 4-0 or 5-0 Supramyd. Thinner sutures tend to erode out of the sclera. Colored sutures are easier to locate in reoperations than white ones.

The assistant provides exposure and steadies the globe, using the bridle sutures adjacent to the break. He also holds back Tenon's capsule with a blade or Schepens retractor. The surgeon further immobilizes the globe by grasping the tendon of a rectus muscle (Fig. 7-11). It is easier to stabilize the globe if the suture needle moves away from, rather than toward, the tendon grasped. Therefore, if a double-armed suture is used, both bites are made from anterior to posterior (Fig. 7-12). An added benefit of this technique is that the suture is tied posteriorly, where Tenon's capsule is thicker; late erosion of the suture is therefore less likely.

It is difficult to place deep scleral sutures in a hypotonous eye without accidental perforation of the choroid. If the eye is soft, the assistant must increase the pressure to a nearly normal level by gentle indentation. If the break is located under a rectus muscle, the assistant can aid in the placement of sutures by retracting the muscle with a muscle hook. Alternatively, the muscle can be temporarily disinserted. Finally, a circumferential explant can be used instead of a radial one because the sutures can then be placed to either side of the muscle.

Scleral bites should be both deep and long so that the suture will not erode out of the sclera postoperatively. A spatula needle must be used. Its tip is introduced slowly into the sclera. When the proper depth has been reached, the needle is carefully pushed along between scleral lamellae (Fig. 7-13*A*). Proper depth can be verified by gently lifting the needle while keeping it parallel to the sclera (Fig. 7-13*B*). The needle must not be allowed to lose its depth (Fig. 7-13*C*), because it is difficult and dangerous to regain depth once it has been

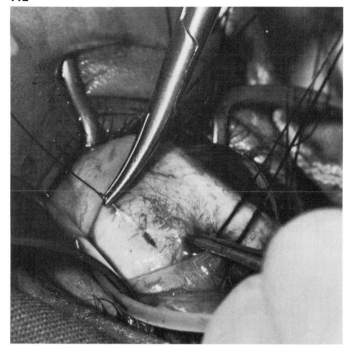

FIG. 7-11. Placement of a scleral suture for a circumferential buckle. The assistant provides exposure and stability by means of two bridle sutures and a retractor. The surgeon further steadies the eye by grasping a rectus muscle tendon with a toothed forceps.

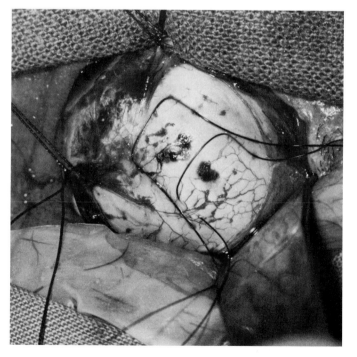

FIG. 7-12. Double-armed sutures placed anterior to posterior in preparation for a silicone sponge. The anterior horns and apex of the flap tear have been localized with diathermy. (For purposes of illustration, the diathermy marks have been darkened with methylene blue.)

lost. When the bite has been completed, the surgeon should push the needle through to its hub and remove it following the curve of the needle. If the spatula needle is twisted during this maneuver, the sharp edge may cut through the choroid and cause bleeding. It may also cut into the overlying sclera and weaken it.

Radial Explants

The explant should extend 1 to 2 mm. beyond the margins of the break. A 5-mm. sponge adequately closes a break 3 mm. wide. If perfectly placed, it can close a break 4 mm. wide. A 7.5-mm. sponge closes breaks 5 to 6 mm. wide. Larger breaks require two sponges placed side by side. Cutting a sponge in half lengthwise reduces its bulk without decreasing the width of the explant (Fig. 7-14). Adequate indentation can still be obtained. The arms of the suture are placed 2 to 3 mm. farther apart than the width of the sponge, e.g., for a trimmed 5-mm. sponge, the sutures are placed 7 mm. apart; for a trimmed 7.5-mm. sponge, 9 to 10 mm. apart. One suture suffices for a small break. For larger breaks, two are needed (Fig. 7-12). To prevent the fishmouth phenomenon (see page 129), the surgeon should begin the posterior bite at the level of the apex of the tear and carry it 3 mm. posteriorly. The anterior suture starts 2 mm. anterior to the horns of the tear. Finally, the tighter the sutures are tied, the higher the indentation of the buckle.

Radial explants are preferred over circumferential explants for closing wide horseshoe tears because they cause much less fishmouthing of the posterior edge.[22, 29] They are also recommended for the treatment of very posterior breaks because it is easier to place the sutures for them than for circumferential explants.

Segmental Circumferential Explants

A segmental circumferential explant is indicated for wide retinal breaks (80°–90°), for multiple breaks at different distances from the ora serrata (Fig. 7-15),[1] and for detachments in which no break is found. The width of the explant depends on the anterior–posterior *length,* not width, of the break. The sutures are asymmetrically placed so that the break will lie on the crest or anterior slope of the buckle. The posterior bite of the mattress suture usually must be made 3 to 4 mm. posterior to the localizing mark of the apex of the tear. If no break has been found, the explant must buckle the posterior vitreous base and must extend the length of the detachment. If the explant encounters a rectus muscle, it must be placed under, not over, the muscle.

IMPLANTS

An implant is a foreign material placed within the sclera to obtain a buckling effect. Its insertion necessitates a lamellar scleral dissection procedure. To insure proper closure of retinal breaks, the scleral bed of the lamellar dissection should extend 3 to 4 mm. beyond each edge of the break or breaks. A circumferential incision is made through the most posterior localization mark on the sclera (Fig. 7-16). Gentle cutting strokes are used. The surgeon spreads the wound frequently with a lateral movement of the blade to avoid cutting too

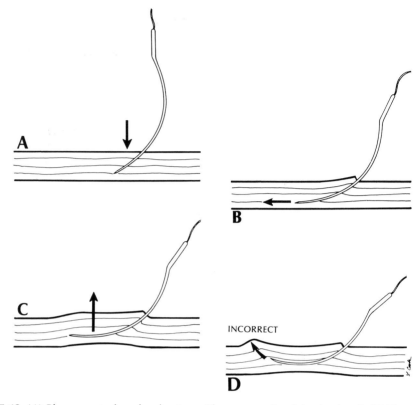

FIG. 7-13. (*A*) Placement of a scleral suture. The proper depth is obtained. (*B*) The needle is guided between the scleral lamellae. (*C*) The surgeon keeps the needle point between the lamellae while lifting the needle gently to verify its depth. (*D*) If the surgeon brings the needle point up prematurely, he loses depth.

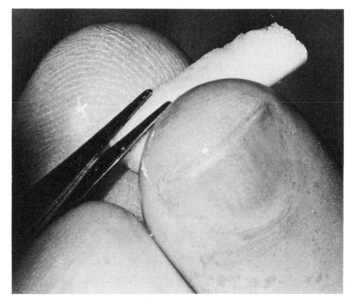

FIG. 7-14. The sponge is cut in half lengthwise to reduce its bulk.

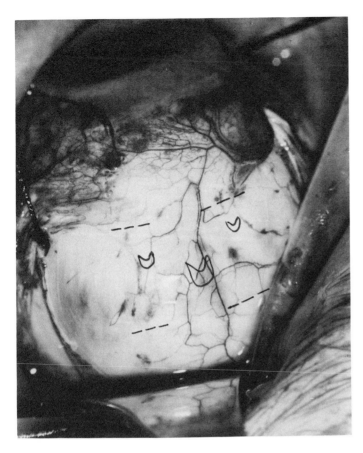

FIG. 7-15. Three retinal breaks at different levels. A circumferential explant is required. Broken lines indicate location of mattress sutures.

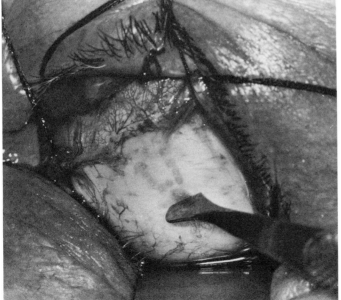

FIG. 7-16. Lamellar scleral dissection. A circumferential incision is made through the most posterior localization mark.

deeply. As soon as the blue color which denotes the choroid is seen through the remaining scleral layers, adequate depth has been reached. The scleral bed must be of even thickness throughout. To this end, a scraping, rather than a cutting, motion is used to *separate* adjacent scleral lamellae. Traction on the scleral flap facilitates the dissection (Fig. 7-17).

Vortex veins are sometimes encountered when the retinal breaks are posteriorly located. While the vortices should be preserved if at all possible, the surgeon should not compromise posterior dissection if it is necessary to seal a break. One or two vortices can be sacrificed if necessary, especially in younger individuals. Elderly patients and high myopes are more prone to complications such as choroidal bleeding and anterior segment necrosis. The extrabulbar portion of the vein to be sacrificed is first carefully cauterized with diathermy. The intrascleral branches are cauterized next. Repeated diathermy as the dissection continues usually prevents bleeding.

After the anterior flap has been dissected, the blunt conical electrode is used to apply staggered rows of diathermy lesions in the scleral bed (Fig. 7-18). The power of the diathermy instrument should be set so that a short application of the electrode results in slight scleral shrinkage and dessication. Too high a setting unnecessarily destroys tissues. If the surgeon prefers cryotherapy, he must apply it before the bed is dissected, or he may penetrate the thin sclera with the probe. If a permanent indentation by an implant is desired, an encircling procedure is necessary (see below).

EXPLANTS VERSUS IMPLANTS

Both implants and explants are effective in producing a high, permanent scleral buckle.[37] Each has advantages and disadvantages.

Advantages of Explants over Implants.

The major advantage of explants is that scleral dissection is not required. Therefore, operating time is decreased, reoperations can be performed with little risk of scleral rupture, and infections are unlikely to penetrate the sclera and lead to endophthalmitis.[25] Also, late intrusions of silicone buckling materials into the eye are extremely rare.

Advantages of Implants over Explants.

In placing an explant suture, it is possible to accidentally perforate the sclera. This has the serious possible complications of subretinal hemorrhage (if the suture is being placed under detached retina) or retinal perforation, occasionally accompanied by vitreous loss (if the suture is being placed under attached retina). Another disadvantage of explants is their higher rate of late extrusion: They are held in place by scleral sutures alone, whereas implants are covered by a scleral layer. At times, explants are cosmetically displeasing (Fig. 7-19).

ENCIRCLING PROCEDURES

Vitreous traction can be reduced permanently by a silicone band or sponge which encircles and constricts the eye. Encircling is indicated when there is

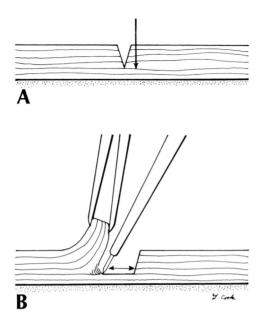

FIG. 7-17. Correct technique for lamellar scleral dissection. (*A*) The surgeon cuts down vertically until the blue color which denotes the choroid is seen. (*B*) Traction on the scleral flap facilitates the dissection. A scraping, not cutting, motion is used.

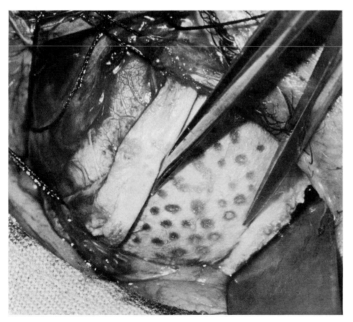

FIG. 7-18. The scleral bed extends 4 mm. posterior to the tear. Adequate diathermy has been applied.

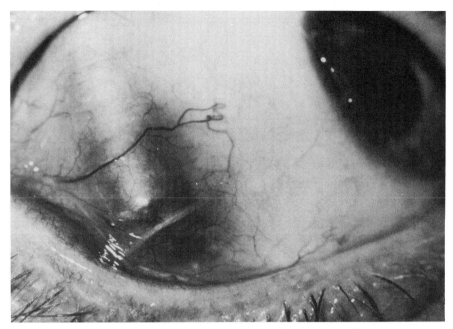

FIG. 7-19. Thin conjunctiva overlying circumferential sponge.

FIG. 7-20. (*A*) Retinal detachment with signs of early massive periretinal proliferation: an equatorial retinal fold (*closed arrow*); a posteriorly rolled edge of the retinal break (*open arrow*), and strong transvitreal traction (*large arrows*). An encircling procedure is indicated. (*B*) The radial sponge and encircling band have relieved enough vitreous traction to permanently close the break.

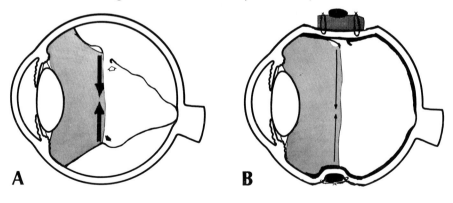

A   B

evidence of early massive periretinal proliferation (MPP), such as fixed folds, retinal tears with posteriorly rolled edges, or equatorial traction folds (Fig. 7-20). It is generally used in the treatment of aphakic retinal detachments because of their high incidence of MPP. It is also used to treat detachments in which no breaks have been found. Care must be taken not to pull the band too tight, or the patient may suffer severe pain, intrusion of the band, or anterior segment necrosis. In most cases, an indentation of 1 mm. suffices to release vitreous traction, but a higher buckle of 2 to 3 mm. is required in the treatment of MPP.

Maximal reduction of vitreous traction can be achieved only if the encircling band constricts the posterior vitreous base. In the presence of strong vitreous traction, this area can be located by an equatorial fold or by a row of small flap tears. Otherwise, the surgeon should place the encircling band 3 to 4 mm. from the ora serrata, where the posterior vitreous base is generally located. The band can be anchored to the sclera by mattress sutures (Fig. 7-21), or by belt loops (Fig. 7-22).

Small breaks (1 to 2 mm. in diameter) can be closed by a 2 mm. wide No. 40 band. The breaks must lie on the crest and anterior slope of the band. Therefore, the anterior bite of the scleral suture is placed at the level of the localization mark. When additional width is required to close a large break, a solid silicone or sponge explant is placed under the encircling band. For multiple breaks at different levels, a segmental circumferential explant or a lamellar scleral dissection with implant can be combined with an encircling band. Alternatively, the eye can be encircled with a 4 mm. band, or with a 5- or 7.5-mm. sponge.

If the encircling procedure has been elected to treat a detachment in which no holes have been found, cryotherapy must be applied to the vitreous base over the length of the detached retina.

DRAINAGE OF SUBRETINAL FLUID

COMPLICATIONS

Drainage should be avoided unless necessary for surgical success[3, 21, 22, 28] because its complications result in redetachment in 1 to 2 per cent of the cases in which it is performed.[16, 29] In many more patients, it is responsible for a permanent decrease in visual acuity. The four major complications of the drainage perforation are choroidal bleeding, retinal incarceration, loss of formed vitreous, and retinal perforation. Choroidal bleeding may result when vessels are lacerated by the drainage perforation. High myopes, elderly patients, and patients with Ehlers-Danlos syndrome are particularly prone to this complication. If blood accumulates under the fovea, the eye almost never regains good visual acuity (Fig. 7-23). Both retinal incarceration and loss of formed vitreous can cause macular pucker or retinal folds, which may keep adjacent breaks open (Fig. 7-24). Vitreous loss is further complicated by a high incidence of massive periretinal proliferation (MPP).[16] Retinal perforation by the drainage instrument usually does not cause postoperative visual loss, but it does require treatment and buckling of the iatrogenic hole.

INDICATIONS FOR USE

Despite its complications, drainage of subretinal fluid must be performed in some cases. Eyes with poor retinal circulation, staphylomatous sclera, or re-

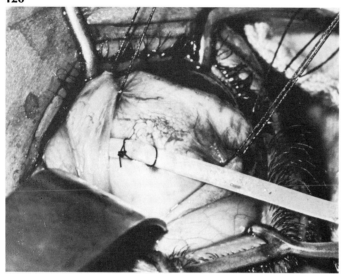

FIG. 7-21. Silicone encircling band anchored to the sclera by a mattress suture. The sutures are tied and cut before drainage.

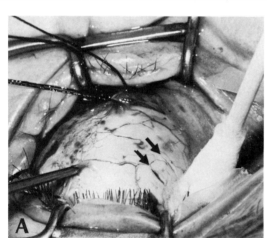

FIG. 7-22. (A) Attaching an encircling band with belt loops. Two 3 mm. grooves (*arrows*) are made 2.5 mm. apart. (B) A number 66 Beaver blade makes a small tunnel between the grooves. (C) Encircling band held in place by belt loop.

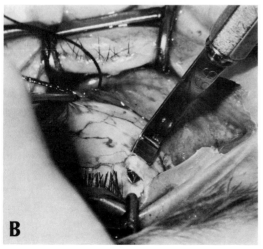

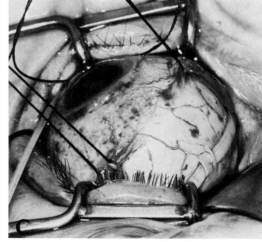

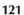

FIG. **7-23.** Large subretinal hemorrhage from the drainage site. The visual acuity is counting fingers.

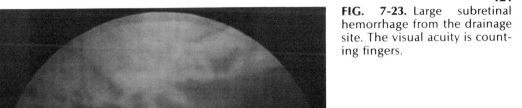

FIG. 7-24. Incarceration of the retina into a drainage perforation. Resultant retinal folds can keep adjacent breaks open.

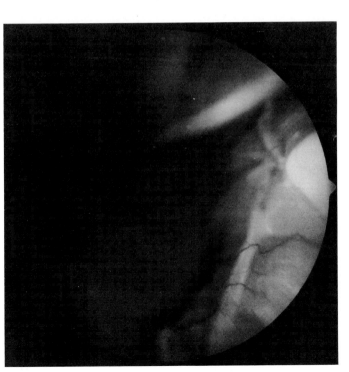

cent intraocular surgery require a drainage procedure because the indentation of the scleral buckle causes a rise in intraocular pressure which could close the central retinal artery or rupture the globe. Drainage of the fluid softens the eye and allows it to accommodate the indentation without a precipitous rise in pressure. Because of their poor outflow facility, glaucomatous eyes also require a drainage procedure; without it, they may sustain damage before their pressure has returned to normal. Eyes with high myopia, senile choroidopathy, or longstanding retinal detachment tend to absorb fluid poorly and should therefore be treated with a drainage procedure.[33] When the retinal break cannot be closed at surgery and it is apparent that vitreous traction (as in MPP or diabetic traction detachment) will prevent postoperative settling of the retina, the subretinal fluid should be drained. Finally, drainage of the subretinal fluid is indicated in cases of retinal detachment with giant tear because such detachments usually do not settle with bed rest and because space must be created for the intraocular gas or air often used in their therapy.

Although Lincoff[22, 23] and others [3, 28, 36] feel that most other cases can be managed without drainage of subretinal fluid, the majority of retinal surgeons choose to drain in a high percentage of their cases. The reason for this is that non-drainage procedures have a lower initial rate of reattachment and a concomitantly higher rate of reoperation.[4, 22] Common causes of failure in non-drainage procedures are inadequate indentation, inaccurate placement of the scleral buckle, vitreous traction, meridional folds, and fishmouthing. Although the reoperation is usually successful, [4, 21, 22] it has its own complications. First of all, should drainage be required, the inflammation caused by the initial operation increases the likelihood of choroidal bleeding from the drainage perforation. Second, postoperative explant infection and extrusion are more common following reoperation.[9] In addition, the patient again faces the danger of anesthesia and the psychic trauma of surgery, as well as having his hospital stay lengthened. Finally, some patients refuse the reoperation.

TECHNIQUE

Since there are few large choroidal blood vessels just above or below the medial or lateral rectus muscle (Fig. 7-25) and under the superior or inferior rectus muscles, these are prime drainage sites. The chances of hemorrhage are further minimized if the choroid is perforated anteriorly. It is best to drain through sclera which will be buckled by the intended implant or explant; then, should the retina be perforated or incarcerated at the drainage site, the repair will not entail placing additional sutures in a soft eye. Drainage under a large bulla of subretinal fluid allows a good quantity of fluid to drain before the retina settles over the drainage site and closes it. It is also important that there be adequate subretinal fluid under the drainage site to avoid retinal perforation by the drainage needle. Two final considerations in selecting a drainage site are (1) that a possible hemorrhage from a nasal perforation is less likely to reach the fovea than is bleeding from a temporal site and (2) that the stiff retina of a fixed fold will rarely incarcerate.

Once the drainage site has been selected, transillumination can be used to locate large choroidal blood vessels (Fig. 7-26).[11] This is especially helpful if

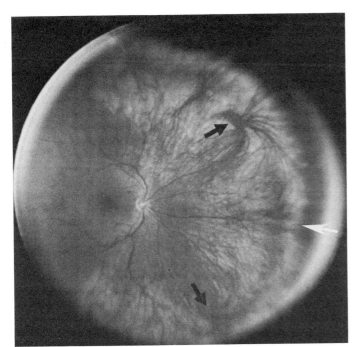

FIG. 7-25. Vortex vein ampullae (*black arrows*) and large choroidal veins are rarely found just above or below the horizontal meridian, which is marked by the long ciliary nerve (*white arrow*).

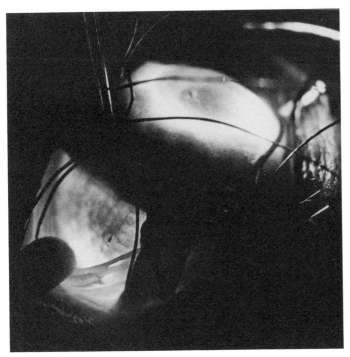

FIG. 7-26. Transillumination of the globe verifies that no large choroidal vessels cross the drainage site.

the drainage site is located posteriorly. The surgeon must be very careful with the occasional rhegmatogenous retinal detachment with shifting fluid. The fluid may move away from the selected drainage site and the retina may be perforated accidentally.

Best drainage is obtained if no scleral fibers overlie the choroid at the drainage site. In a lamellar dissection procedure, a radial cut-down to the choroid is made through the prepared lamellar bed. If fluid must be drained outside of the bed, or if an explant is to be used, the choroid is exposed in the bed of a small triangular scleral flap (Fig. 7-27*A*) or simply through a radial cut-down. A longer cut-down provides better exposure, allowing safe removal of the deep scleral fibers. The thicker the sclera, the longer the cut-down necessary. If the drainage site is made in a lamellar bed, no suture is needed to close it. If it will be under an explant, the scleral flap or cut-down is closed with a preplaced absorbable suture. If the drainage site will not be covered by an implant or an explant, it should be closed with a preplaced non-absorbable suture. In order to reduce the possibility of hemorrhage, the exposed choroid is treated with several applications of low-intensity diathermy. The blunt conical electrode is used (Fig. 7-27*A*).

It is important that the eye be normotensive for drainage. If the intraocular pressure is too high, it must be lowered by acetazolamide, mannitol, or by an anterior chamber paracentesis. Otherwise, when the choroid is perforated, sudden decompression can cause choroidal hemorrhage or rapid evacuation of the subretinal fluid followed by retinal or vitreous incarceration. If the intraocular pressure is too low, the assistant should indent the eye with a cotton-tipped applicator to restore the pressure to nearly normal. The choroid is then perforated with the diathermy needle electrode (Fig. 7-27*B*), a 27-gauge hypodermic needle, a tapered suture needle, or a Zeigler knife (Fig. 7-27*C*). Prior to the perforation, the surgeon must verify that the pressure in the eye is not elevated. A gentle thrust to a depth of 1 mm. is sufficient to perforate.

When the subretinal fluid begins to drain, gentle indentation of the globe opposite the drainage site helps to shift subretinal fluid toward it. Excessive pressure on the eye to force subretinal fluid out may cause retinal incarceration and must be avoided. Traction on the edge of the scleral flap with a small forceps helps to hold the sclera and choroid away from the retina, reducing the chances of incarceration (Fig. 7-27*B*).

When little or no subretinal fluid remains, a small hemorrhage or pigment granules usually appear at the drainage site. At this time, the fundus must be inspected to see if there is subretinal fluid over the drainage site. If there is, gentle lateral traction on the scleral flap may allow further drainage. Occasionally, another choroidal perforation is required. It is almost never necessary to drain until all of the subretinal fluid is gone or even until the break is flat on the buckle, as long as the buckle is properly placed and of adequate height. When enough fluid has been drained, the suture over the drainage site is tied immediately (Fig. 7-28). This prevents retinal incarceration, which might otherwise result from a sudden elevation in intraocular pressure owing to manipulation of the globe. If the perforation site is in a lamellar dissection bed, the scleral flap suture closest to it is immediately closed for the same reason.

FIG. 7-27. (A) Drainage of sub-retinal fluid in an explant procedure. The choroid is exposed in the bed of a small triangular scleral flap and is treated with multiple applications of low-intensity diathermy using the blunt conical electrode. (B) Perforation of the choroid with the needle electrode. The needle enters the eye tangentially to reduce the possibility of retinal perforation. A suture is preplaced for closing the scleral flap after drainage. During drainage, the surgeon pulls outward on the flap to prevent retinal incarceration. (C) Drainage in the bed of an implant procedure. The choroid is perforated with a Ziegler knife.

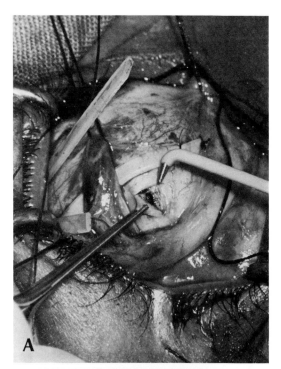
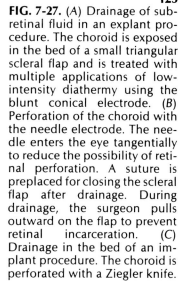

A

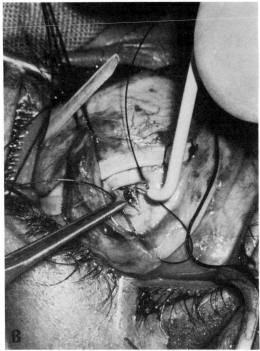

B

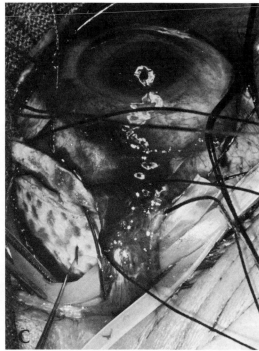

C

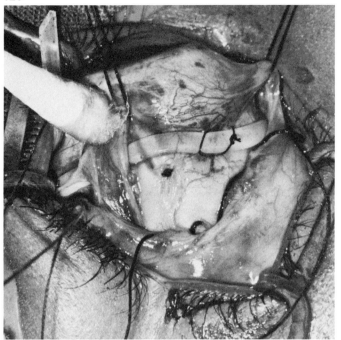

FIG. 7-28. The scleral flap is closed immediately after drainage.

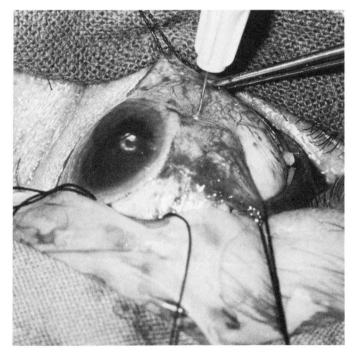

FIG. 7-29. Air injection through the pars plana 4 mm. from the limbus. A 30-gauge needle is used.

INTRAVITREAL INJECTIONS

AIR

Tamponade of a retinal break with air temporarily closes a break as effectively as a scleral buckle. The choroid/pigment epithelium then absorbs the subretinal fluid, effecting contact between the treated retinal pigment epithelium and the sensory retina. Intraocular air is also useful in closing giant tears or, as mentioned below, tears showing the fishmouth phenomenon. It can also be used in the treatment of retinal detachment with macular holes (see chapter 8, Surgery of Complicated Cases).

In some cases in which drainage of subretinal fluid is attempted near large tears, liquid vitreous can pass through the tear and out of the eye through the drainage site. The eye becomes very soft, but the amount of fluid under the retina remains the same. In these cases, the surgeon should close the drainage site, place the scleral buckle, and inject air to tamponade the retinal hole. Once the hole has been so closed, the subretinal fluid is absorbed.

Sterile air can be obtained by drawing room air through a millipore filter. After the filter is removed, the air is injected into the vitreous cavity through a 30-gauge needle. Intravitreal injections are made through the pars plana 4 mm. from the surgical limbus (Fig. 7-29). It is very important that a sharp needle be used and that the needle have passed through the nonpigmented epithelium of the pars plana prior to the injection. This must be confirmed by indirect ophthalmoscopy. As the air is injected, the assistant monitors intraocular pressure to prevent excessive injection.

Hemorrhage from such injections is very rare but can occur. Of course, the surgeon must be very careful not to strike the lens with the needle as it enters the eye. If the needle does not pass cleanly through the pars plana epithelium before the air is injected, a dialysis may occur. If too much air is injected, the excessive rise in intraocular pressure may occlude the central retinal artery, incarcerate the retina in a drainage site, rupture the globe through a weakened area, or tear out scleral sutures. Although fibrous ingrowth through the site of penetration is very rare, it may occur.

INERT GASES

Inert gases such as sulfur hexafluoride (SF_6)[8, 17, 27, 30] and octofluorocyclobutane (C_4F_8)[17, 30] offer two major advantages over the use of room air for intravitreal injection. First, they expand postoperatively, as nitrogen and oxygen diffuse from surrounding tissues into the gas bubble. Within the first 24 to 48 hours, SF_6 expands to twice its initial volume. Even after drainage of subretinal fluid, a high scleral buckle may reduce the volume of the vitreous cavity, limiting the space which an air bubble can occupy. If SF_6 is used, a small amount of gas injected at surgery can still result in a final air bubble large enough to tamponade the retinal break. No more than 1.5 cc. of pure SF_6 should be used; otherwise, expansion of the gas bubble can raise the intraocular pressure high enough to close the central retinal artery. If the proper amount is used, enough fluid leaves the eye through the trabecular meshwork to compensate for the expansion of the gas. The second advantage of the inert gases is that they remain in the eye for 11 to 14 days. Thus, the treated sensory retina and pigment epithelium are kept in contact for a longer period of time, allowing a firmer adhesion to develop.

When nitrous oxide is being used for anesthesia, the surgeon must monitor the intraocular pressure closely and should avoid injection of a large volume of sulfur hexafluoride. Nitrous oxide rapidly diffuses into the injected gas bubble and may cause a precipitous elevation of the intraocular pressure.[12]

INTRAOPERATIVE PROBLEMS

RETROBULBAR HEMORRHAGE

If, after retrobulbar anesthesia, the eye becomes rock-hard owing to an expanding hemorrhage in the closed orbital space, the surgeon must act immediately to avoid retinal artery occlusion. He decompresses the orbit by a lateral canthotomy[19] and by a rapid 360° peritomy. This is a rare complication of retrobulbar anesthesia.

SMALL PUPIL

If the pupil will not dilate preoperatively, a sector iridectomy can be performed just prior to the retinal detachment surgery. Xenon or argon photocoagulation can also be used to widen the pupil. Several small burns 2 mm. from the pupil will shrink the iris and enlarge the pupil.

CORNEAL OPACIFICATION

Corneal transparency may be decreased by contact with the solutions used for sterile preparation of the operative field. Excessive scleral depression during localization or treatment may cause epithelial edema. A clearer view of the fundus can be obtained if the cloudy corneal epithelium is removed with a rounded blade. The epithelium usually heals postoperatively in 1 to 2 days, but healing may take longer in diabetics.

POSTERIOR EXPOSURE

It is sometimes difficult to place sutures for posteriorly located breaks. Adequate exposure is usually provided by a lateral canthotomy. If this does not suffice, disinsertion of a rectus muscle may be necessary. A traction suture placed through the stump of the muscle enables the surgeon to manipulate the eye in order to obtain the desired exposure.

STAPHYLOMA

Placing sutures into very thin sclera is dangerous because the choroid may accidentally be perforated. Moreover, the sutures may pull out postoperatively. The scleral sutures should be placed in adjacent thicker sclera. Since the mattress suture is then wider than actually required, one must use a larger explant than is needed to close the break (Fig. 7-30). Silicone sponges are less likely to intrude into the eye through thin sclera than are solid silicone explants. When a true staphyloma exists, the surgeon must be very careful not to raise the intraocular pressure too high during the procedure, or the globe may rupture.

INADVERTENT PERFORATION OF THE GLOBE

If the needle accidentally perforates the choroid while sutures are being placed, subretinal fluid may drain, causing hypotony. The suture should be removed and its replacement suture positioned so that the accidental drainage site will later fall under the buckle. Pressure with a cotton-tipped applicator over the accidental drainage site may make the eye firm enough for proper placement of the remaining sutures. If too much fluid has drained, even this will not suffice, and an intraocular injection of saline solution will be necessary to restore the intraocular pressure. If a deep suture perforates attached retina, the area should be treated with cryotherapy and scleral buckling.

INCREASED INTRAOCULAR PRESSURE

As the surgeon ties the scleral sutures, he must constantly monitor the intraocular pressure. An estimate can be obtained by palpation ("finger tension") or by indentation with a muscle hook. More accurate readings can be taken with the Shiotz or Perkins tonometers. If the pressure is high, the surgeon should inspect the optic disc to see if the central retinal artery is either pulsating or occluded. If the media are hazy, the best way to confirm arterial patency is to induce pulsations while pressing gently on the eye. If pulsations cannot be produced, the artery may be occluded.

If, during the tying of the scleral sutures, the central retinal artery is occluded or in danger of occluding, the surgeon must lower the intraocular pressure before tying the rest of the sutures. He can try several maneuvers. If the eyelids have been pushed behind the globe, decreasing the available orbital space, they should be pulled forward and the globe reposited. In phakic patients, an anterior chamber paracentesis is helpful. This is not advised for aphakic eyes, because vitreous may become incarcerated in the wound. If these measures are insuffient, the surgeon can loosen some of the sutures or decrease the constriction of the encircling band if it has already been tied. A last resort is vitreous aspiration.

THE FISHMOUTH PHENOMENON

Scleral buckling may result in a meridional fold formed by redundant retina on the posterior slope of the buckle (Fig. 7-31). The buckle, in this case, actually prevents reattachment. It keeps the break open and allows a free passage of subretinal fluid posteriorly. This phenomenon, called "fishmouthing," is more likely to occur with circumferential than with radial buckling. If the break is superiorly located, an intravitreal injection of air may close it. If the superior break remains open or if the break is inferior, the meridional folding can be reduced by decreasing the height of the buckle (by loosening

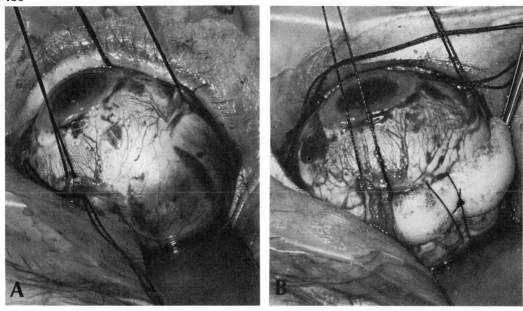

FIG. 7-30. (*A*) Staphylomatous sclera in which sutures for a radial explant cannot be placed. (*B*) Circumferential 7.5 mm. sponge anchored by a mattress suture placed in thicker sclera anterior and posterior to the staphyloma.

FIG. 7-31. The fishmouth phenomenon. (*A*) Flap tear in detached retina. Solid line indicates width of the tear. (*B*) A circumferential buckle (between arrows) compresses the tear (large line indicates original width), keeping its posterior edge open.

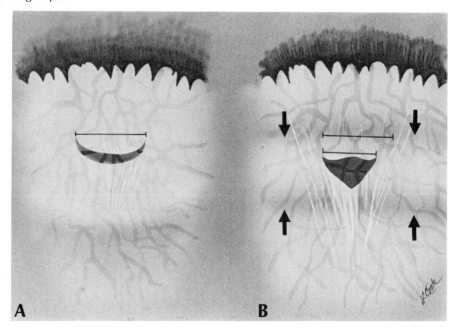

the sutures). Alternatively, a radial element can be placed under and perpendicular to the circumferential buckle.

CLOSING

After he has drained the subretinal fluid, the surgeon ties the sutures holding the explant(s) (Fig. 7-32) or those closing the scleral flaps over the implant (Fig. 7-33). If the surgeon is not certain that he has correctly localized the break, he can use slipknots to facilitate later repositioning of the buckle. If an encircling band is being used, it is tightened at this time and the ends are tied together (Fig. 7-34). The surgeon must avoid excessive tightening of the encircling band. An indentation of 1 to 2 mm. is usually sufficient.

If all of the subretinal fluid has been drained, it is easy to determine if the scleral buckle has been correctly placed. If subretinal fluid remains under the hole, the surgeon can push gently on the scleral buckle while observing the retinal break with the indirect ophthalmoscope. The increased indentation helps him to assess the buckle's relationship to the break.

When an implant is being used and the buckle has not been placed far enough posteriorly, it is necessary to dissect farther back and to use a larger implant than previously intended. If a segmental circumferential explant is not properly placed anteriorly or posteriorly, the surgeon can replace the original suture with a correctly located one. Finally, if the posterior edge of an encircling explant is near to, but not fully buckling, the hole, a trimmed piece of sponge can be slipped under the encircling band perpendicular to it. This technique is particularly helpful when there is fishmouthing of the posterior edge of the break.

It is important not to trim a radial explant until adequate closure of the retinal break has been confirmed. If the explant has not been properly placed posteriorly or anteriorly, an additional suture can easily be placed. If a radial sponge has not been placed in the proper radial meridian, it is necessary to replace the original mattress suture. Usually it is best to place the new scleral suture(s) prior to removing the old one(s). This will maintain the intraocular pressure until the new suture(s) can be safely placed.

When it has been ascertained that the scleral buckle has been properly placed (Fig. 7-35), that no drainage site complications have occurred, and that the intraocular pressure is not unduly elevated, a culture is taken. Antibiotic solutions reduce the bacterial count; they may either be used to irrigate the orbit or they may be injected into Tenon's capsule. Explants should be covered by a thick layer of Tenon's capsule to prevent late extrusion. To this end, Tenon's capsule is pulled up and anchored to the tendon of the rectus muscle in each quadrant (Fig. 7-36). The conjunctiva is closed with plain catgut suture (Fig. 7-37). Atropine and antibiotic ointment are then applied, and the eye is patched with a semipressure dressing to reduce postoperative eyelid edema.

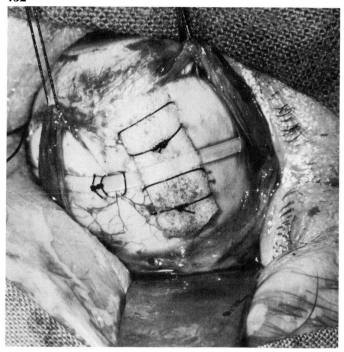

FIG. 7-32. Silicone sponge sutured to the sclera. In this case, an encircling band was also used.

FIG. 7-33. (*A*) A solid silicone implant (grasped with forceps) is placed in the bed of the dissection. In this case, an encircling silicone band (*arrow*) is also used. It fits into a groove in the implant. (*B*) Scleral flaps are closed with mattress sutures.

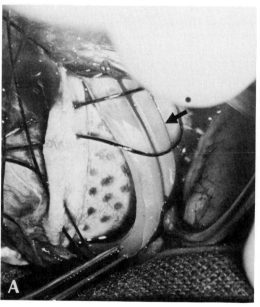

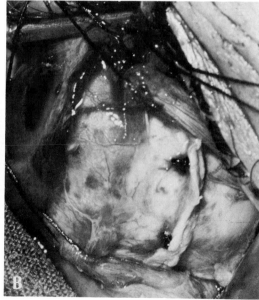

FIG. 7-34. The encircling band is tied after its tension has been adjusted.

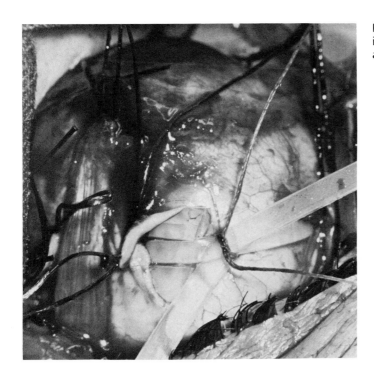

FIG. 7-35. Postoperative photograph of flap tear correctly placed on the scleral buckle (in stereo).

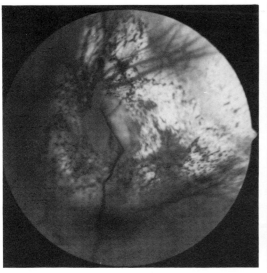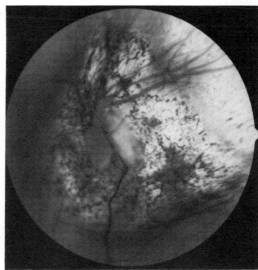

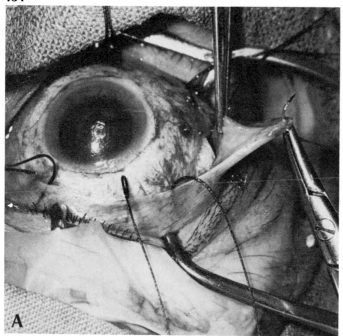

FIG. 7-36. (*A*) A toothed forceps grasps Tenon's capsule.

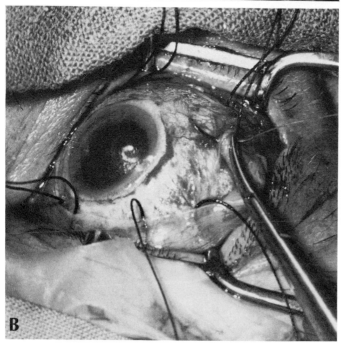

(*B*) Tenon's capsule is anchored to the tendon of all four rectus muscles.

FIG. 7-37. (*A*) The ends of a relaxing incision are brought together.

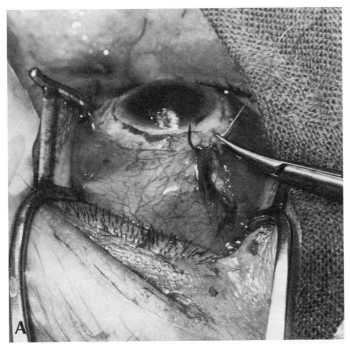

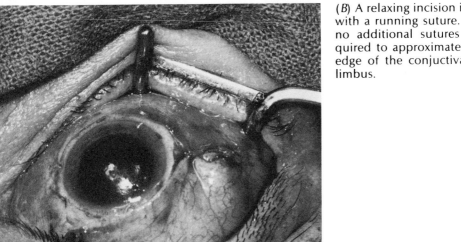

(*B*) A relaxing incision is closed with a running suture. Usually no additional sutures are required to approximate the cut edge of the conjuctiva to the limbus.

REFERENCES

1. **Aaberg, TM, Wiznia RA:** The use of solid soft silicone rubber exoplants in retinal detachment surgery. Ophthalmic Surg 7:98, 1976
2. **Blodi FC:** Injection and impregnation of liquid silicone into ocular tissues. Am J Ophthalmol 71:1044, 1974
3. **Chignell AH:** Retinal detachment surgery without drainage of subretinal fluid. Am J Ophthalmol 77:1, 1974
4. **Chignell AH, Fision LG, Davies EWG, Hartley RE, Gundry MF:** Failure in retinal detachment surgery. Br J Ophthalmol 57:525, 1973
5. **Cibis PA:** Vitreoretinal Pathology and Surgery in Retinal Detachment. St. Louis, CV Mosby, 1965, pp 199–249
6. **Cibis PA:** Vitreous cavity and retinal detachment. Mod Probl Ophthalmol 5:59, 1967
7. **Cockerham WD, Schepens, CL, Freeman HM:** Silicone injection in retinal detachment. Arch Ophthalmol 83:704, 1970
8. **Fineberg E, Machemer R, Sullivan P, Norton EWD, Hamasaki D, Anderson D:** Sulfur hexafluoride in owl monkey vitreous cavity. Am J Ophthalmol 79:67, 1975
9. **Flindall RJ, Norton EWD, Curtin VT, Gass JDM:** Reduction of extrusion and infection following episcleral silicone implants and cryopexy in retinal detachment surgery. Am J Ophthalmol 71:835, 1971
10. **Freeman HM, Hawkins WR, Schepens CL:** Anterior segment necrosis, an experimental study. Arch Ophthalmol 75:644, 1966
11. **Freeman HM, Schepens CL:** Innovations in the technique of drainage of subretinal fluid: transillumination and choroidal diathermy. Trans Am Acad Ophthalmol Otolaryngol 78:829, 1974
12. **Fuller D, Lewis ML:** Nitrous Oxide anesthesia with gas in the vitreous cavity. Am J Ophthalmol 80:778, 1975
13. **Havener WH, Gloeckner S:** Atlas of Diagnostic Techniques and Treatment of Retinal Detachment. St. Louis, CV Mosby, 1967, pp 108–118
14. **Hilton GF:** Subretinal pigment migration. Effects of cryosurgical retinal reattachment. Arch Ophthalmol 91:445, 1974
15. **Holekamp TLR, Arribas NP, Boniuk I:** Bupivacaine anesthesia in retinal detachment surgery. Arch Ophthalmol 97:109, 1979
16. **Humphrey WT, Schepens CL, et al:** The release of subretinal fluid and its complications. In Pruett RC, Regan CDJ (eds): Retina Congress. New York, Appleton-Century-Crofts, 1972 pp 383–390
17. **Kelley FP, Edelhauser HF, Aaberg TM:** Intraocular sulfur hexafluoride and octofluorocyclobutane. Arch Ophthalmol 96:511, 1978
18. **King LM, Schepens CL:** Limbal peritomy in retinal detachment surgery. Arch Ophthalmol 91:295, 1974
19. **Kraushar MF, Seelenfreund MH, Freilich DB:** Central retinal artery closure during orbital hemorrhage from retrobulbar injection. Trans Am Acad Ophthalmol Otolaryngol 78:65, 1974
20. **Laqua H, Machemer R:** Repair and adhesion mechanisms of the cryotherapy lesion in experimental retinal detachment. Am J Ophthalmol 81:833, 1977
21. **Leaver PK, Chignell AH, Fison LG, Payne JR, Saunders SH:** Role of non-drainage of subretinal fluid in reoperation for retinal detachment. Br J Ophthalmol 59:252, 1975
22. **Lincoff H:** Should retinal breaks be closed at the time of surgery? In Brockhurst RJ, Boruchoff SA, Hutchinson BT, Lessell S (eds): Controversy in Ophthalmology. Philadelphia, WB Saunders, 1977, pp 582–598
23. **Lincoff H, Kreissig I:** The treatment of retinal detachment without drainage of subretinal fluid. Trans Am Ophthalmol Otolaryngol 76:1221, 1972
24. **Lincoff H, Kreissig I:** Advantages of radial buckling. Am J Ophthalmol 79:955, 1975
25. **Lincoff H, Nadel A, O'Connor P:** The changing character of the infected scleral implant. Arch Ophthalmol 84:421, 1970
26. **Norton EWD:** The present status of cryotherapy in retinal detachment surgery. Trans Am Acad Ophthalmol Otolaryngol 73:1029, 1969

27. **Norton EWD:** Intraocular gas in the management of selected retinal detachments. Trans Am Acad Ophthalmol Otolaryngol 77:85, 1973

28. **O'Connor PR:** Absorption of subretinal fluid after external scleral buckling without drainage. Am J Ophthalmol 76:30, 1973

29. **Okun E:** Discussion of Lincoff H, Kreissig I: The treatment of retinal detachment without drainage of subretinal fluid. Trans Am Acad Ophthalmol Otolaryngol 76:1232, 1972

30. **Peyman GA, Vygantas CM, Bennett TD, Vygantas AM, Brubaker S:** Octofluorocyclobutane in vitreous and aqueous humor replacement. Arch Ophthalmol 93:514, 1975

31. **Pruett RC:** The fishmouth phenomenon. II. Wedge scleral buckling. Arch Ophthalmol 95:1782, 1977

32. **Ramsay RC, Knobloch WH:** Ocular perforation following retrobulbar anesthesia for retinal detachment surgery. Am J Ophthalmol 86:61, 1978

33. **Robertson DM:** Delayed absorption of subretinal fluid after scleral buckling procedures. Am J Ophthalmol 87:57, 1979

34. **Schepens CL:** Current management of retinal detachment: progress or chaos? Ann Ophthalmol 3:21, 1971

35. **Schwartz A, Rathbun E:** Scleral strength impairment and recovery after diathermy. Arch Ophthalmol 93:1173, 1975

36. **Scott JD:** Retinal detachment surgery without drainage. Trans Ophthalmol Soc UK 90:57, 1970

37. **Stone RD, Irvine AR, Santos E:** An ultrasonographic study of the persistence of buckle height three years after segmental sponge explants. Am J Ophthalmol 84:508 1977

8

SURGERY
OF
COMPLICATED
CASES

MACULAR HOLES

A macular hole is responsible for 0.5 to 0.7 per cent of retinal detachments.[6, 11] In most cases, the hole is caused by either very high myopia or trauma.[11]

In many retinal detachments caused by peripheral breaks, accumulation of intraretinal fluid may result in a foveal "cyst" with extremely thin walls. Even with the aid of fluorescein angiography and biomicrosopy, the most experienced examiner may be unable to differentiate such a "cyst" from a full-thickness macular hole.[1, 11] For this reason alone, all peripheral breaks must be closed before a suspected macular hole is treated (Fig. 8-1). Moreover, if even an unequivocal full-thickness macular hole is accompanied by any peripheral breaks, these breaks should be closed first. This often cures the detachment, even though the macular hole has not been treated (Fig. 8-2).[11] If all of the peripheral breaks have been treated and the detachment persists, or if there are no accompanying peripheral breaks, the macular hole must be treated. Three treatment techniques are discussed below, in ascending order of complexity.

TREATMENT 1: CRYOTHERAPY AND DRAINAGE

In many cases, a combination of cryotherapy (or diathermy) and drainage of subretinal fluid will close the hole and cure the detachment.[6] This technique is most successful for detachments which have no vitreous traction, provided the eye has no significant posterior staphyloma (Fig. 8-3). If the vitreous is adherent to the posterior retina, vitreous traction will redetach the retina before a firm chorioretinal scar can develop (Fig. 8-4). If retinal shrinkage (a result of early massive periretinal proliferation) has taken place, the detached retina cannot stretch enough to settle into a large posterior staphyloma (Fig. 8-5).

In a non-buckling procedure such as this, the injection of air or gas into the vitreous cavity performs some of the functions of a scleral buckle. It insures total absorption of the subretinal fluid and keeps the retina in contact with the treated choroid long enough to allow the scarring process to begin. In cases with little subretinal fluid, the injection of air or gas also substitutes for a drainage procedure.[13] Postoperatively, the patient is positioned face down so that the air rises against the retina, tamponading the hole (Fig. 8-6). The subretinal fluid is then absorbed, and the subsequent chorioretinal scar prevents redetachment. If there is a large accumulation of subretinal fluid, it must be drained in order to make room for sufficient air or gas. SF_6 is preferred to air because the SF_6 remains in the eye long enough to allow a firm chorioretinal scar to develop.

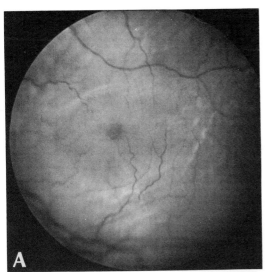

FIG. 8-1. (*A*) Temporal retinal detachment with a very thin macula. Clinically, the patient was thought to have a full-thickness macular hole. (*B*) Fluorescein angiogram. Increased transmission of background fluorescence through the macula is consistent with the misdiagnosis of full-thickness macular hole. (*C*) A peripheral retinal break was found and closed. The retina is reattached. Visual acuity is 6/15 (20/50). No macular hole is present. Normal fluorescein angiogram.

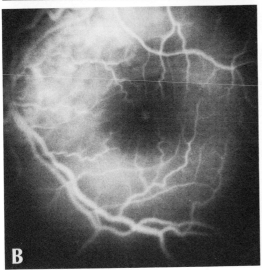

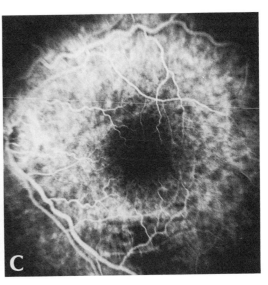

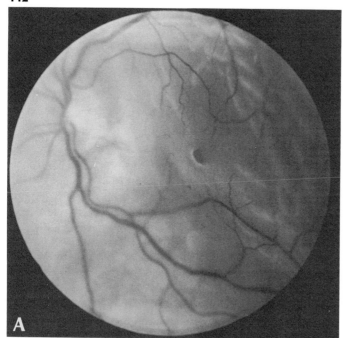

FIG. 8-2. (*A*) Retinal detachment with full-thickness macular hole.

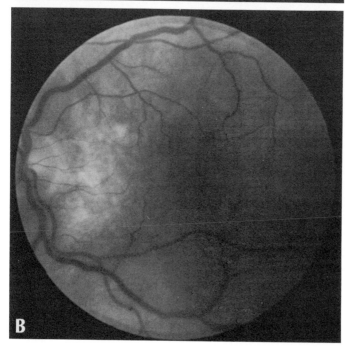

(*B*) Peripheral breaks were closed by a scleral buckling procedure. The retina is reattached, even though the macular hole has not been treated.

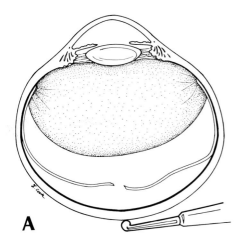

A

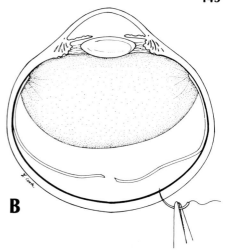

B

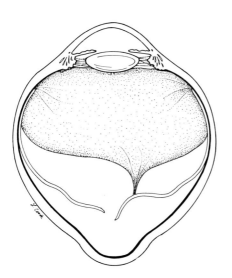

FIG. 8-4. Cryotherapy and drainage alone will fail if there is sufficient posterior vitreous traction to redetach the retina before a firm chorioretinal scar develops.

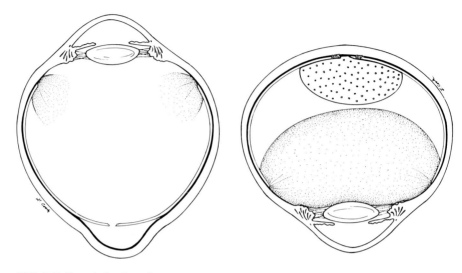

FIG. 8-5. Top, left. Cryotherapy and drainage alone will fail if a shunken retina cannot settle into a large posterior staphyloma.

FIG. 8-6. Top, right. An intravitreal air injection will tamponade the macular hole, allowing absorption of subretinal fluid.

FIG. 8-7. Bottom, left. Removal of the formed vitreous by vitrectomy permits the injection of a larger volume of air or sulfur hexafluoride. The macular hole may be sealed in spite of a posterior staphyloma.

FIG. 8-8. Bottom, right. A macular buckle flattens the posterior staphyloma.

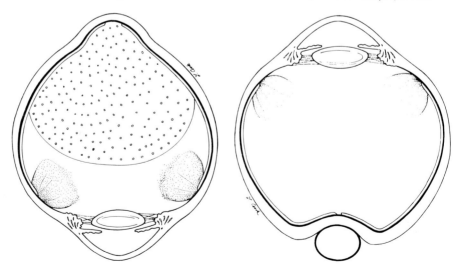

The complications of drainage, cryotherapy, diathermy, and gas injection have already been discussed (see chapter 7, Basic Surgical Technique). Additional risks are involved in the treatment of macular holes. The drainage site in these cases is usually located posteriorly, so there is a high risk of perforating a large choroidal vessel. Moreover, choroidal hemorrhage from the drainage site is more common in high myopia than in emmetropia, and therefore much more common in cases with macular hole. Finally, in applying cryotherapy to the macula, the surgeon runs the risk of accidentally freezing the optic nerve and causing blindness.

TREATMENT 2: VITRECTOMY

The above procedures will not reattach the macula if there is vitreous traction on the posterior retina (Fig. 8-4). After vitrectomy has released the traction,[7] cryotherapy and air or gas combine to close and seal the hole. Removal of the formed vitreous also permits injection of a larger volume of air or gas. With proper positioning of the patient, the air or gas keeps the retina in contact with the treated choroid for a longer period of time and may effect a cure even in cases of posterior staphyloma (Fig. 8-7).

TREATMENT 3: SCLERAL BUCKLING PROCEDURE

If the retina has shrunk (as in early massive periretinal proliferation) and cannot stretch enough to settle into a posterior staphyloma, a scleral buckling procedure is required to indent the staphyloma enough to allow reattachment of the retina (Fig. 8-8).[15]

Placement of a local macular buckle has many complications.[12] Because it is difficult to achieve adequate exposure of the macula, especially in elongated, highly myopic eyes, the choroid can be perforated while posterior scleral sutures are being placed for an explant; a subretinal or vitreous hemorrhage can result. When a scleral bed is being prepared for an implant, short ciliary arteries can be transected or the globe perforated.

These complications can be avoided by a sling procedure (Figs. 8-9 and 8-10), which eliminates the placement of sutures in the macular area.[4,12] A silicone band or sponge anchored anteriorly is run along an arc of a great circle of the eye and under the macula. In order to make room for adequate indentation, the subretinal fluid may be drained or the liquid vitreous aspirated. A drawback of the sling procedure is that it distorts a large area of the retina. Its most serious complication is possible compression of the optic nerve and concomitant severe loss of vision.

GIANT TEAR WITH ROLLED-OVER RETINA

There are two major problems in the treatment of giant tears (circumferential tears 90° or larger) with rolled-over retina (Fig. 8-11): first, initially unrolling the retina, and second, keeping it unrolled while cryosurgical or diathermy scarring takes place. Vitrectomy can solve both of these problems.[9] The patient is placed on a Stryker frame to permit later repositioning. Generally,

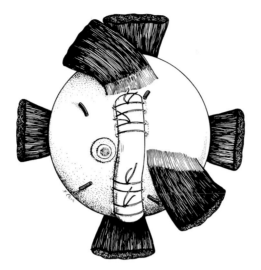

FIG. 8-9. A sling procedure buckles the macular hole.

FIG. 8-10. Macula buckled by the sling technique (Stereo).

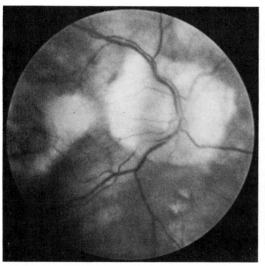 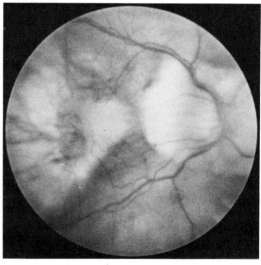

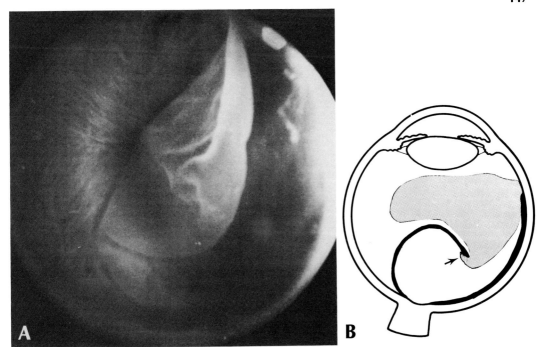

FIG. 8-11. (*A*) Giant tear with rolled-over retina. (Courtesy L. K. Sarin, M.D.) (*B*) Frequently, the vitreous is adherent to the anterior retina (*arrow*) and overlies the posterior surface of the retina, making it very difficult for the surgeon to unroll the retina.

lensectomy is required to allow removal of all of the anterior vitreous. Once the formed vitreous has been removed, the retina is unrolled by the vitrectomy instrument and a bent needle or by an intraocular balloon.[5] The patient is then positioned so that the retina continues to unroll while the vitreous contents are being replaced entirely with a 40:60 mixture of SF_6:air (Fig. 8-12). Postoperatively, the patient is positioned so that the gas holds the retina in place (Fig. 8-13).

MASSIVE PERIRETINAL PROLIFERATION

In advanced cases of MPP (see chapter 2, Pathophysiology), a scleral buckling procedure alone cannot reattach the retina. Vitrectomy is required to release the vitreous traction, which will otherwise keep the retinal breaks open, and to remove the preretinal membranes which stiffen and shrink the retina. The vitrectomy instrument is used to cut transvitreal membranes, and a bent needle is used to peel preretinal membranes from the retinal surface.[8] These techniques release the traction and restore enough retinal flexibility to allow anatomic reattachment of 36 per cent of retinal detachments judged inoperable without vitrectomy.[10]

Because it is often difficult to assess the severity of MPP, and because vitrectomy is a relatively hazardous procedure, the surgeon should attempt a

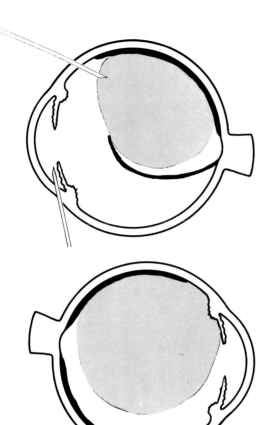

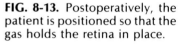

FIG. 8-12. After lensectomy and vitrectomy, the patient is positioned so that the rolled-over retina is dependent. Then, as the injected gas bubble expands, it pushes the retina back into position. A needle in the anterior chamber drains liquid from the eye.

FIG. 8-13. Postoperatively, the patient is positioned so that the gas holds the retina in place.

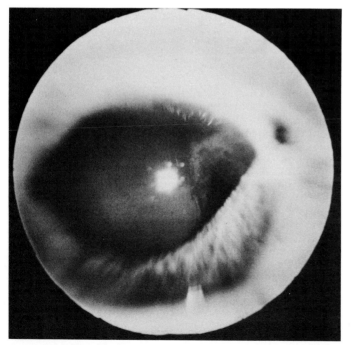

FIG. 8-14. Pars plana epithelium dragged toward cataract wound by incarcerated vitreous.

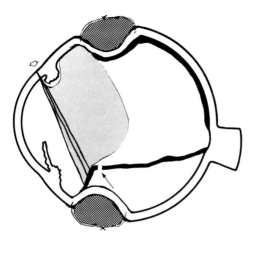

FIG. 8-15. Aphakic retinal detachment with vitreous incarcerated in the cataract wound (*open arrow*). Strong vitreous traction prevents settling of the retinal break (*arrow*) on the scleral buckle.

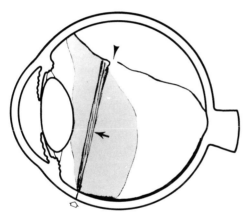

FIG. 8-16. Retinal tear (*arrowhead*) and detachment caused by fibrovascular tissue (*arrow*) proliferating through the entry wound (*open arrow*) of a foreign body.

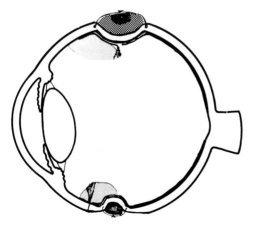

FIG. 8-17. After the fibrous tissue has been cut by vitrectomy, the detachment is cured by an encircling procedure.

scleral buckling procedure first, unless he is certain that the MPP is too far advanced for this to succeed. If this initial surgery fails, vitrectomy and a second scleral buckling procedure are the only recourse.

APHAKIC RETINAL DETACHMENT WITH VITREOUS TRACTION

Traction on the retina caused by vitreous incarceration in a cataract wound (Fig. 8-14) sometimes prevents reattachment of an aphakic retinal detachment by a scleral buckling procedure (Fig. 8-15).[14] The traction must be released by vitrectomy before the retina can be successfully reattached.

PENETRATING INJURIES

A late complication of penetrating injury is the proliferation of episcleral fibrovascular tissue into the eye along the path of the foreign body (Fig. 3-3). The vitreous fibers act as a scaffold upon which the tissue grows. When the fibrovascular membrane contracts, it can cause a retinal tear 90° to 180° from the site of penetration (Fig. 8-16). The resultant retinal detachment can often be repaired by a scleral buckling procedure, but vitrectomy is indicated when traction prevents the retina from settling.[2, 3] Scissors must be used if the vitrectomy instrument cannot cut the dense fibrovascular tissue. Often the traction can be released by peeling the dense membrane from the retina with a bent needle. The vitrectomy instrument then removes the membrane from the eye and an encircling scleral buckling procedure is performed (Fig. 8-17). Even with the aid of vitreous surgery, the prognosis for these cases remains poor.

PROLIFERATIVE DIABETIC RETINOPATHY

Vitreous traction associated with proliferative diabetic retinopathy may cause a non-rhegmatogenous traction retinal detachment. If the macula is detached or is likely to detach, vitrectomy is performed to release the traction.

In some cases, the traction causes breaks (see chapter 3, Predisposing Conditions). Management of rhegmatogenous retinal detachment with a strong traction component is very difficult. Occasionally, a high scleral buckle can be used in conjunction with an encircling band to both close the break and release some of the traction. Scleral shortening procedures may allow the retina to flatten out. Vitrectomy offers the possibility of releasing all of the traction. Once this has been achieved, a standard scleral buckling procedure has a much greater chance of success. No matter what therapy is attempted, less than 50 per cent of the cases can be repaired.

REFERENCES

1. **Adams ST:** Retinal detachment due to macular and small posterior holes. Arch Ophthalmol 66:528, 1961
2. **Benson WE, Machemer R:** Severe penetrating injuries treated with pars plana vitrectomy. Am J Ophthalmol 81:728, 1976

3. **Cox MS, Freeman HM:** Retinal detachment due to ocular penetration. Arch Ophthalmol 96:1354, 1978

4. **Feman SS, Hepler RS, Straatsma BR:** Rhegmatogenous retinal detachment due to macular hole. Arch Ophthalmol 91:371, 1974

5. **Freeman HM:** Vitreous surgery. X. Current status of vitreous surgery in cases of rhegmatogenous retinal detachment. Trans Am Acad Ophthalmol Otolaryngol 77:202, 1973

6. **Howard GM, Campbell CJ:** Surgical repair of retinal detachments caused by macular holes. Arch Ophthalmol 81:317, 1969

7. **Machemer R, Norton EWD:** A new concept for vitreous surgery. 3. Indications and results. Am J Ophthalmol 74:1034, 1972

8. **Machemer R:** A new concept for vitreous surgery. 7. Two-instrument techniques in pars plana vitrectomy. Arch Ophthalmol 92:1340, 1976

9. **Machemer R, Allen AW:** Retinal tears 180° and greater. Management with vitrectomy and intravitreous gas. Arch Ophthalmol 94:1340, 1976

10. **Machemer R, Laqua H:** A logical approach to the treatment of massive periretinal proliferation. Ophthalmology 85:584, 1978

11. **Margherio RR, Schepens CL:** Macular breaks. 1. Diagnosis, etiology, and observations. Am J Ophthalmol 74:219, 1972

12. **Margherio RR, Schepens CL:** Macular breaks. 2. Management. Am J Ophthalmol 74:233, 1972

13. **Norton EWD:** Intraocular gas in the management of selected retinal detachments. Trans Am Acad Ophthalmol Otolaryngol 77:85, 1973

14. **Norton EWD, Machemer R:** New approach to the treatment of selected retinal detachments secondary to vitreous loss at cataract surgery. Am J Ophthalmol 72:705, 1971

15. **Schepens CL, Okamura ID, Brockhurst RJ:** The scleral buckling procedures. I. Surgical techniques and management. Arch Ophthalmol 58:797, 1957

9

POSTOPERATIVE MANAGEMENT

ROUTINE CASES

Postoperatively, the patients are mobilized as quickly as possible. Hair brushing and washing, as well as shaving and bathing, are permitted. However, if there is air or sulfur hexafluoride in the vitreous cavity, the patient is kept on bed rest, positioned so that the gas rises against the break to tamponade it. The eye which has had surgery is patched; bilateral patches are occasionally used after non-drainage procedures to facilitate settling of the retina. Atropine (1%) solution is instilled twice daily and an antibiotic–corticosteroid mixture instilled three times daily. The severity of postoperative pain varies widely. Many patients are comfortable with mild analgesics. Others require strong, even intramuscular, analgesics, especially after lengthy procedures.

The patients are discharged on the 3rd or 4th postoperative day with instructions to return in 1 week for a follow-up examination. At this time all but the most strenuous activities are permitted.

POSTOPERATIVE INTRAOCULAR PRESSURE

Patients who have had retinal detachment surgery must be watched carefully for glaucoma.[47] The postoperative intraocular pressure should be measured by applanation tonometry, in preference to Schiotz tonometry, because scleral buckling procedures decrease scleral rigidity.[46] In these patients, Schiotz tonometry readings average 6 to 9 mm. Hg lower than applanation tonometry readings.

A frequent side benefit of scleral buckling procedures is a permanent decrease in intraocular pressure caused by decreased aqueous secretion. Friedman studied twelve patients with bilateral glaucoma and unilateral retinal detachment.[23] Postoperatively, glaucoma therapy was unnecessary in eleven of the eyes which had had retinal detachment surgery, whereas all of the eyes which had not had surgery still required treatment for glaucoma.

THE EARLY COMPLICATIONS

ANGLE CLOSURE GLAUCOMA

Following 1 per cent of scleral buckling procedures, choroidal congestion causes a forward displacement of the ciliary body and closure of the filtration angle.[47] The congestion may result from a tight encircling band, a large scleral dissection, or excessive cryotherapy or diathermy. The consequent increased intraocular pressure causes pain and corneal edema. This condition may not be identified, because the central portion of the anterior chamber may remain deep. The diagnosis is made by applanation or Mackay-Marg tonometry and gonioscopy. Because pupillary block is not a contributing factor, treatment with pilocarpine and/or iridectomy is not effective. Proper management includes the use of acetazolamide and, if necessary, mannitol. Frequent applications of topical corticosteroids may help to prevent peripheral anterior synechiae. If the pressure remains elevated, the encircling band must be loosened or removed.

SYMBLEPHARON

The eye must be inspected carefully for adhesions between the bulbar and palpebral conjunctiva, especially after a lateral canthotomy has been performed. Early adhesions can be broken with a glass rod or a cotton-tipped applicator.

ANTERIOR SEGMENT NECROSIS

A number of the procedures involved in retinal repair can occlude blood vessels and cause anterior segment necrosis. Diathermy can occlude the long ciliary arteries.[20] Tenotomy of three or more rectus muscles can occlude the anterior ciliary arteries.[24, 25] If several vortex veins are occluded, e.g., by a tight, posteriorly located encircling band or by a broad lamellar dissection, anterior segment necrosis can result.[32] Patients with poor circulation may suffer anterior segment necrosis from scleral buckling over the long ciliary arteries.[49]

Radial or segmental circumferential explants can also interfere with anterior segment circulation. Iris fluorescein angiography performed on consecutive cases in which explants had been used showed a high percentage of filling defects in the quadrant of the iris corresponding to the location of the explant.[18]

In severe cases, the earliest finding is striate keratopathy. Later there is corneal edema without elevated intraocular pressure. Many patients have marked chemosis. White flakes floating in the anterior chamber or deposited on the lens are diagnostic of the condition. Large keratitic precipitates may be present. Late findings are hypotony due to atrophy of the ciliary processes, irregularly dilated pupil, iris atrophy, posterior synechiae, and cataract (Fig. 9-1). Histologically, there is necrosis of the iris and ciliary body, thrombosis of the major arterial circle of the iris, and necrosis of the choroid under implants.[7, 17]

Although clinically significant anterior segment necrosis is rare, many patients who have had retinal surgery show some evidence of damage to the anterior segment circulation or innervation. A transient increase in corneal thickness is common.[19] Corneal sensitivity is often abnormal for 3 to 6 months.[11] Abnormalities can occur in both the parasympathetic[40] and the sympathetic[37] innervation of the pupil. If anterior segment necrosis is suspected,

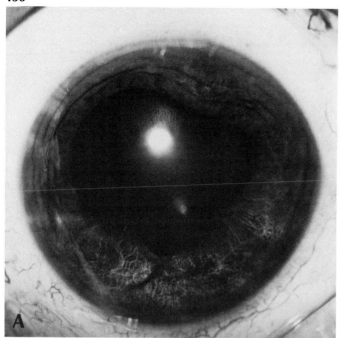

FIG. 9-1. (*A*) Iris atrophy and posterior synechiae following moderately severe anterior segment necrosis.

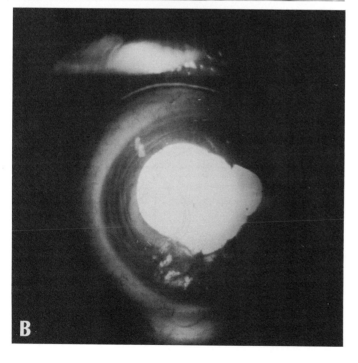

(*B*) Transillumination defects in the inferior half of the atrophic iris.

the patient should be treated with high doses of topical and systemic corticosteroids, and the encircling band, if present, should be loosened.

Patients with sickle cell disease are especially prone to this condition. Preventive measures to be considered in their treatment are avoidance of encircling procedures, exchange transfusion,[51] and hyperbaric oxygenation.[22]

INFECTION

Unusually severe pain is an early indicator of orbital infection. Early signs are marked chemosis and injection of the conjunctiva. Mucopurulent discharge follows. Some patients have numerous inflammatory cells in the vitreous. A localized exudate over a scleral buckle is a particularly ominous sign, for it may indicate early scleral necrosis and endophthalmitis. The most common bacteria involved are Staphylococcus aureus, Pseudomonas, and Proteus. The infection cannot be cured by antibiotics alone; the implant or explant must be removed. Most studies indicate that 20 to 30 per cent of retinas will detach following removal of the scleral buckle.[39, 52, 56, 61] In more recent studies, however, only 4 to 13 per cent redetached.[319, 34] Cases which are least likely to redetach are those with little vitreous traction and those in which the buckle has been in place for a month or more. If the retina does redetach, a reoperation can be performed 1 week after removal of the buckle, by which time the orbit will have resterilized itself.

CHOROIDAL DETACHMENT

Choroidal detachments are quite common after retinal detachment surgery, especially in elderly or aphakic patients. They are also seen in patients with broad or posteriorly located buckles and in patients who have undergone reoperations. Prolonged hypotony after drainage of subretinal fluid is felt to be a contributing factor, although choroidal detachments have also been reported following non-drainage procedures.[12] Choroidal detachments cannot be prevented by subconjunctival depot corticosteroids.[10]

The choroidal fluid characteristically accumulates during the first 3 to 4 days after surgery and then remains stable for 1 to 2 weeks. Because of decreased aqueous secretion, the intraocular pressure remains low despite apparent occlusion of the filtration angle.

Treatment is rarely indicated, even if large choroidal detachments meet in the center of the vitreous cavity. In almost all cases, they will spontaneously reabsorb, and the retinal surfaces will not remain adherent to each other.

PIGMENT FALLOUT

Cryotherapy shatters pigment epithelial cells, releasing pigment into the subretinal space.[2] The pigment accumulates in the most dependent part of the retinal detachment. In limited retinal detachments, the pigment collects at the junction of attached and detached retina, causing a "pseudo-demarcation line" (Fig. 9-2).[57] If the detachment is total, pigment may collect in the posterior pole. Hilton has shown that such a pigment accumulation does not cause a decrease in visual function.[33]

LATE COMPLICATIONS

REFRACTIVE ERROR

Encircling procedures usually cause a slight increase in myopia.[27] Non-encircling scleral buckling procedures may cause regular astigmatism. Sometimes irregular astigmatism which cannot be corrected by spectacles is seen after placement of a radial explant.[8] Many patients have decreased accommodation, which may persist for several months.

STRABISMUS

Excessive traction on and freezing of[3] the extraocular muscles contribute to transient postoperative diplopia. Permanent diplopia may result from disinsertion of a rectus muscle, but it is more common if the disinserted muscle is a vertical rectus, rather than a horizontal one.[35] It may also occur following the placement of a large implant or explant under a rectus muscle.[54,55] Excessive scarring following reoperations can also cause permanent diplopia.

Since most patients recover completely, it is advisable to wait at least 6 months before considering corrective muscle surgery. It is then important to determine whether the diplopia is caused by scar tissue preventing rotation of the eye or by the underaction of a muscle which is bound down to the globe. Forced ductions aid greatly in this determination.[48] When the limitation in motility is caused by scar tissue, the eye cannot be forcibly rotated away from the apparently overacting muscle. To restore ocular motility, the surgeon must first dissect the scar tissue from the sclera. Tenon's capsule and the conjunctiva are then recessed to the level of the muscle insertion. Anteriorly, the sclera is left bare.[48] When the limitation is caused by underaction of a muscle adherent to the globe, the eye can be forcibly rotated in all directions. The adherent muscle must be freed and resected.[48]

EXTRUSION OF IMPLANTS OR EXPLANTS

Pain, mucopurulent discharge, and subconjunctival hemorrhage may be signs of an extruding explant or implant. In many patients, initial erosion of the sponge through the conjunctiva is followed by localized infection (Fig. 9-3). Removal of the explant or implant cures the infection. If a sponge explant has been used in addition to an encircling band, it usually suffices to remove the explant alone.[50]

MACULAR PUCKER

Proliferation of a preretinal astrocytic membrane causes crinkling or pucker of the macula (Fig. 9-4) after 9 to 15 per cent of retinal detachment operations.[28,29,30,40,58] Macular pucker is usually first noted 6 to 8 weeks after surgery.

The mechanism which causes pucker is unknown. The condition can occur after an uncomplicated procedure, but its incidence is higher following certain intraoperative complications, such as loss of formed vitreous, retinal in-

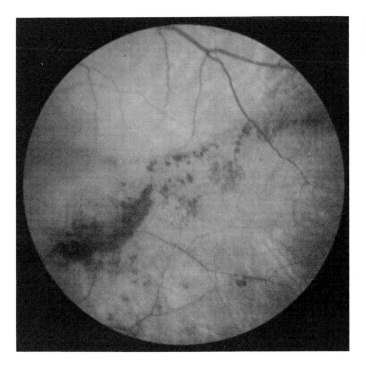

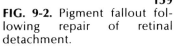

FIG. 9-2. Pigment fallout following repair of retinal detachment.

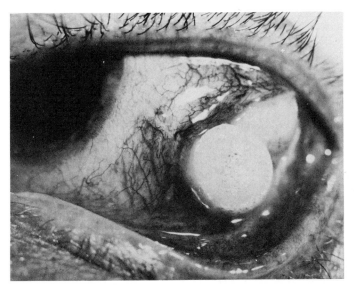

FIG. 9-3. Extruding radial silicone sponge explants.

carceration, subretinal hemorrhage, and vitreous hemorrhage.[58] Some authors have found that it is more common after diathermy procedures than after cryotherapy.[30]

SLOW ABSORPTION OF SUBRETINAL FLUID

Even if all breaks have been closed, it may take weeks for complete absorption of the subretinal fluid following either non-drainage operations or operations in which the subretinal fluid has been incompletely drained (Fig. 9-5).[13, 45, 49a] If the surgeon is confident that no breaks are open, he should wait patiently for all of the fluid to reabsorb. If fluid begins to reaccumulate, exudative retinal detachment, a missed break, or an open break must be ruled out.

POSTOPERATIVE EXUDATIVE RETINAL DETACHMENT

It is important to recognize exudative retinal detachments because they may be confused with reaccumulation of subretinal fluid due to an open break. In exudative detachments, the retinal breaks are successfully closed and remain closed, but 2 or 3 days after surgery fluid from the choroid begins to accumulate posterior to the buckle. The fluid shifts with changes in the position of the eye and is often turbid. Choroidal detachments are frequently present. Spontaneous absorption of the fluid takes up to twelve weeks, but it may be accelerated by systemic corticosteroids.[1]

When an open break is the source of the accumulating subretinal fluid, the fluid is usually clear and does not shift with changes in the position of the eye. Careful examination is necessary to locate the break, which must then be closed by reoperation.

FAILURE TO REATTACH THE RETINA

All surgical failures are caused by an open retinal break. In some cases, photocoagulation or the injection of air or gas can effect a cure; in others, reoperation is necessary. In any case of surgical failure, it is difficult to know whether or not reapplication of cryotherapy or diathermy should be performed as part of the reoperation. If the sensory retina was thoroughly frozen in the first operation, tight junctions will probably form between the pigment epithelium and Müller's cells without retreatment. However, if only the pigment epithelium was frozen in the original operation, retreatment probably is indicated after 4 to 5 days. By this time, the treated pigment epithelium will have been replaced by pigment epithelial cells sliding over from untreated areas, and a firm adhesion will not result.

INADEQUATE ABSORPTION OF THE SUBRETINAL FLUID

If the retinal break is not in contact with the scleral buckle at the end of the surgery, reattachment depends on spontaneous absorption of enough subretinal fluid to lower the break onto the buckle. In some cases, even with a high and properly placed buckle, the surgery will fail from insufficient postopera-

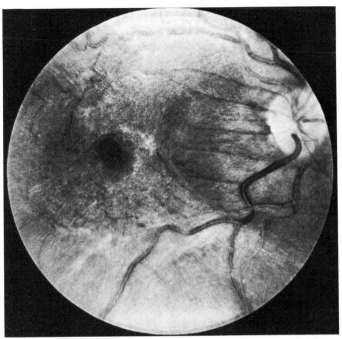

FIG. 9-4. Severe macular pucker. Contraction of the preretinal membrane wrinkles the retina. Notice straightening of the blood vessels between the disc and the fovea.

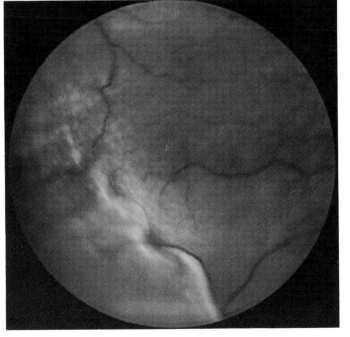

FIG. 9-5. Persistent subretinal fluid 2 months after a scleral buckling procedure which successfully closed the retinal breaks. One month after this photograph was taken, the fluid was absorbed.

tive absorption of fluid. There are two major causes of such failures: First, certain ocular conditions are characterized by a poor absorption capability. High myopia, senile choroidopathy, and longstanding retinal detachment fall into this category. Second, incorrectly assessed vitreous traction can keep the break open and thus prevent the absorption of fluid.[44]

In other cases, a properly positioned scleral buckle can fail to close the break because it does not adequately indent the sclera.[13] In non-drainage procedures, it is often difficult to obtain a high buckle because tightening the scleral sutures may excessively raise the intraocular pressure. A low buckle may not close the break even after partial postoperative absorption of subretinal fluid. If the fluid had been drained, however, even this low buckle would have sufficed to permanently close the break.

If a small amount of fluid separates the retina from the buckle, reoperation may be avoided. Argon laser or xenon arc photocoagulation may seal the break, repairing the detachment.[15]

When too much fluid remains for photocoagulation to form an adequate scar, the patient may be treated with an intravitreal injection of air (or sulfur hexafluoride), provided the break is not inferiorly located. More air can be injected if an anterior chamber paracentesis is also performed. With proper positioning of the patient, the air or gas tamponades the break and usually effects closure and subsequent reabsorption of the subretinal fluid. If it does not, drainage of the fluid is indicated. If this fails to permanently close the break, the original buckle must be replaced by a higher one.

MISPLACED SCLERAL BUCKLE

If the break is not fully closed by the buckle, the operation may fail. The most common error is failure to place the buckle far enough posteriorly. Fluid then leaks down the posterior slope of the buckle, redetaching the retina (Fig. 6-37A). Less common is inadequate anterior support (Fig. 9-6). Fluid then leaks anteriorly, runs along the anterior slope of the buckle, and eventually leaks posteriorly (Fig. 6-37B).

The only remedy for a misplaced scleral buckle is reoperation to correctly position the buckle.

COMPLICATIONS OF THE INITIAL SURGERY

Unrecognized or untreated surgical complications may prevent reattachment of the retina. Retinal incarceration at the drainage site (Fig. 7-24) causes folds which may keep the original break open. Reoperation is necessary to flatten the folds and close the break. Traction from incarcerated vitreous may prevent the retina from settling or may reopen an initially closed retinal break. The traction must be relieved and the break closed by a high encircling buckle. Iatrogenic retinal holes, caused either by the drainage needle or by a deep scleral suture, must be found and buckled. If a large break is kept open by fishmouthing, or a small break is kept open by meridional folding, the case will fail. Corrective measures are discussed in chapter 7.

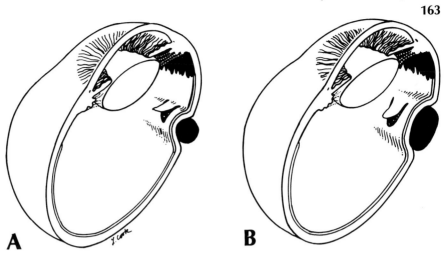

FIG. 9-6. (*A*) Incorrectly buckled flap tear. The break is not supported anteriorly. (*B*) Correctly buckled flap tear. The entire break is supported.

UNDETECTED BREAK

An undetected retinal break may be responsible for surgical failure. If the subretinal fluid has been drained, new fluid will accumulate; if it has not, the retina will not settle. The only remedy is to find and close the break.

VITREOUS TRACTION

If excessive vitreous traction is present, retinal breaks closed at the time of surgery may be reopened in the early postoperative period. On reoperation, a higher scleral buckle, combined with an encircling procedure, is required. In some cases, the traction must be released by vitrectomy.

INADEQUATE CRYOTHERAPY OR DIATHERMY

Fluid can reaccumulate through an initially flat retinal break if the cryotherapy lesions were not contiguous or if the diathermy applications were too weak. Reoperation may be avoided if photocoagulation is performed immediately.

LATE DETACHMENT OF THE RETINA

If an initially reattached retina redetaches after a period of 6 weeks or longer, the case can be considered a late redetachment rather than a surgical failure. Redetachment results from either the development of a new tear, or from the reopening of the original break.

NEW RETINAL TEARS

In a recent series,[60] the most common cause of late redetachment (16 of 19 cases) was a new retinal tear resulting from increased vitreous traction. Of the 16 cases, the new tear was located posterior to an encircling band in 9 (Fig. A-15), on an encircling band in 3, and in previously unbuckled quadrants in 4 (Fig. A-14). The prognosis for successful reattachment is excellent in these cases; 15 of the 16 detachments were repaired. New tears that overlie a buckle can often be closed by photocoagulation alone. Tears in other locations require a segmental scleral buckle and cryotherapy (or diathermy). Since a new break may signify early MPP, an encircling band is used in cases not previously encircled (Fig. A-14).

REOPENING OF THE ORIGINAL BREAK

Increased Vitreous Traction

Extension of a Flap Tear. Increased vitreous traction on a flap tear can extend the tear through an area of cryotherapy, allowing anterior leakage of subretinal fluid.[5,16] This problem can be avoided if the cryotherapy of flap tears is extended to the ora serrata. If this has not been done initially and detachment results, photocoagulation may close the break. Otherwise it is necessary to apply additional cryotherapy or diathermy. If the increased traction has extended the tear beyond the original scleral buckle, a broader buckle must be substituted at the time of supplemental treatment.

Massive Periretinal Proliferation (see Chapter 2, Pathophysiology). MPP is the most common cause of failure of initial retinal detachment surgery, but is an uncommon cause of late redetachment. If mild MPP reopens the original break, repair can often be effected by a higher scleral buckle used in combination with an encircling procedure. Reapplication of cryotherapy or diathermy is also required. More advanced cases necessitate vitrectomy (see chapter 8, Surgery of Complicated Cases).

Decreased or Displaced Scleral Buckle

Change in Height or Position of the Buckle. Occasionally a suture erodes out of the sclera. This may either decrease the height of the buckle or cause it to shift its position. Vitreous traction can then reopen the retinal break. Most of these redetachments can be cured by repeating the original operation.

Removal of the Scleral Buckle. The scleral buckle must be removed if it is responsible for late infection[28,50,60] or severe postoperative pain, or if it extrudes through the conjunctiva. As noted above, removal of this support will lead to redetachment in 4 to 30 per cent of the cases.[34,39,56,60] If the retina redetaches immediately, the reoperation must be delayed 1 week after removal of the buckle to allow the orbit to resterilize itself.

PROGNOSIS AND VISUAL RESULTS

ANATOMIC REATTACHMENT

With current techniques, 90 to 95 per cent of detached retinas can be repaired.[9, 26, 43] Success rates for different types of retinal detachment vary as follows:

1. Excellent prognosis (nearly 100 per cent):
   Detachments due to dialysis[31] or to small or round holes[4]
   Detachments with demarcation lines[6]
   Detachments with minimal subretinal fluid.
2. Slightly poorer prognosis (85 to 95 per cent):
   Aphakic detachments[9, 44]
   Total detachments, detachments with associated detachment of the non-pigmented epithelium of the pars plana[9]
   Detachments due to flap tears[4]
3. Poor prognosis (30 to 50 per cent):
   Detachments with associated choroidal detachment[9, 25, 53]
   Detachments with breaks larger than 180°[21, 35, 41]
   Detachments with massive periretinal proliferation[41]

POSTOPERATIVE VISUAL ACUITY

Overall, approximately 50 per cent of patients will regain a visual acuity of 6/15 (20/50) or better; 25 per cent, 6/18 to 6/30 (20/60 to 20/100); and 25 per cent, 6/60 (20/200) or worse.[44] Postoperative visual acuity chiefly depends on whether or not and how long the macula was detached before surgery.[28, 29] When the macula has detached, necrosis of photoreceptors may prevent good postoperative visual acuity. Seventy-five per cent of patients with a macular detachment of less than 1 week's duration will obtain a final visual acuity of 6/21 (20/70) or better, as opposed to 50 per cent with a macular detachment of 1 to 8 weeks' duration.[28]

The prognosis for vision is far better in cases in which the macula has not detached, though 15 per cent of them lose vision from macular pucker or cystoid macular edema.[28] Obviously, intraoperative complications also affect the final visual acuity.

REFERENCES

1. **Aaberg TM, Pawlowski GJ:** Exudative retinal detachments following scleral buckling with cryotherapy. Am J Ophthalmol 74:245, 1972
2. **Abraham RK, Shea M:** Cryopexy for improved results in the prophylaxis of retinal detachment. Trans Ophthalmol Soc UK 88:297, 1968
3. **Bell FC, Pruett RC:** Effects of cryotherapy on extraocular muscles. Ophthalmic Surg 8:71, 1977
4. **Benson WE, Morse PH:** The prognosis of retinal detachment due to lattice degeneration. Ann Ophthalmol 10:1197, 1978
5. **Benson WE, Morse PH, Nantawan P:** Late complications following cryotherapy of lattice degeneration. Am J Ophthalmol 84:514, 1977
6. **Benson WE, Nantawan P, Morse PH:** Characteristics and prognosis of retinal detachments with demarcation lines. Am J Ophthalmol 84:641, 1977

7. **Boniuk M, Zimmerman LE:** Pathologic anatomy of complications. In Schepens CL, Regan CDJ (eds.): Controversial Aspects of the Management of Retinal Detachment. Boston, Little, Brown, 1965, p 263

8. **Burton TC:** Irregular astigmatism following episcleral buckling procedures. Arch Ophthalmol 90:447, 1973

9. **Burton TC:** Preoperative factors influencing anatomic success rates following retinal detachment surgery. Trans Am Acad Ophthalmol Otolaryngol 83:499, 1977

10. **Burton TC, Stevens TS, Harrison TJ:** The influence of subconjunctival depot corticosteroid on choroidal detachment following retinal detachment surgery. Trans Am Acad Ophthalmol Otolaryngol 79:845, 1975

11. **Cambiaggi A:** Comment. In Schepens CL, Regan CDJ (eds): Controversial Aspects of the Management of Retinal Detachment. Boston, Little, Brown, 1965, p 224

12. **Chignell AH:** Choroidal detachment following retinal detachment without drainage of subretinal fluid. Am J Ophthalmol 73:860, 1972

13. **Chignell AH, Fison LG, Davies EWG, Hartley RE, Gundry MF:** Failure in retinal detachment surgery. Br J Ophthalmol 57:525, 1973

14. **Chignell AH, Talbot J:** Absorption of subretinal fluid after nondrainage retinal detachment surgery. Arch Ophthalmol 96:635, 1978

15. **Curtin VT, Norton EWD, Gass JDM:** Photocoagulation, its use in prevention of reoperation after scleral buckling procedures. Trans Am Acad Ophthalmol Otolaryngol 71:432, 1967

16. **Delaney WV:** Retinal tear extension through the cryosurgical scar. Br J Ophthalmol 55:205, 1971

17. **Eagle RC, Yanoff M, Morse PH:** Anterior segment necrosis following scleral buckling in hemoglobin SC disease. Am J Ophthalmol 75:426, 1973

18. **Easty DL, Chignell AH:** Fluorescein angiography in anterior segment ischemia. Br J Ophthalmol 57:18, 1973

19. **Fiore JV, Newton JC:** Anterior segment changes following the scleral buckling procedure. Arch Ophthalmol 84:284, 1970

20. **Freeman HM, Hawkins WR, Schepens CL:** Anterior segment necrosis: an experimental study. Arch Ophthalmol 75:644, 1966

21. **Freeman HM, Schepens CL, Couvillion GC:** Current management of giant retinal breaks. Trans Am Acad Ophthalmol Otolaryngol 74:59, 1973

22. **Freilich DB, Seelenfreund MG:** Hyperbaric oxygen for retinal detachment in sickle cell anemia. Arch Ophthalmol 90:90, 1973

23. **Friedman Z, Neumann E:** Effect of retinal detachment surgery on the course of preexisting open-angle glaucoma. Am J Ophthalmol 80:702, 1975

24. **Girard LF, Beltranena F:** Early and late complications of extensive muscle surgery. Arch Ophthalmol 64:576, 1960

25. **Gottlieb F:** Combined choroidal and retinal detachment. Arch Ophthalmol 88:481, 1972

26. **Griffith RD, Ryan EA, Hilton GF:** Primary retinal detachments without apparent breaks. Am J Ophthalmol 81:420, 1976

27. **Grupposo SS:** Visual results after scleral buckling with silicone implant. In Schepens CL, Regan CDJ (eds): Controversial Aspects of the Management of Retinal Detachment. Boston, Little, Brown, 1965, pp. 354–363

28. **Grupposo SS:** Visual acuity following surgery for retinal detachment. Arch Ophthalmol 93:327, 1975

29. **Gundry MF, Davies EWG:** Recovery of visual acuity after retinal detachment surgery. Am J Ophthalmol 77:310, 1974

30. **Hagler WS, Aturaliya U:** Macular pucker after retinal detachment surgery. Br J Ophthalmol 55:451, 1971

31. **Hagler WS, North W:** Retinal dialysis and retinal detachment. Arch Ophthalmol 79:376, 1968

31a. **Hahn YS, Lincoff A, Lincoff H, Kreissig I:** Infection after sponge implantation for scleral buckling. Am J Ophthalmol 87:180, 1979

32. **Hayreh SS, Baines JAB:** Occlusion of the vortex veins: an experimental study. Br J Ophthalmol 57:217, 1973

33. **Hilton GF:** Subretinal pigment migration. Arch Ophthalmol 91:445, 1974
34. **Hilton GF, Wallyn RH:** The removal of scleral buckles. Arch Ophthalmol 96:2061, 1978
35. **Kanski JJ:** Giant retinal tears. Am J Ophthalmol 79:846, 1975
36. **Kanski JJ, Elkington AR, Davis MS:** Diplopia after retinal detachment surgery. Am J Ophthalmol 76:38, 1973
37. **Kronfield PC:** Segmental impairment of pupillary motility after operations for retinal detachment. Trans Am Ophthalmol Soc 59:239, 1961
38. **Leaver PK, Chignell AH, Fison LG, Pyne JR, Saunders SH:** Role of non-drainage of subretinal fluid in reoperation for retinal detachment. Br J Ophthalmol 59:252, 1975
39. **Lincoff H, Nadel A, O'Connor P:** The changing character of the infected scleral implant. Arch Ophthalmol 84:421, 1970
40. **Lobes LA, Burton TC:** The incidence of macular pucker after retinal detachment surgery. Am J Ophthalmol 85:72, 1978
41. **Machemer R, Allen AW:** Retinal tears 180° and greater. Management with vitrectomy and intravitreal gas. Arch Ophthalmol 94:1340, 1976
42. **Machemer R, Laqua H:** A logical approach to the treatment of massive periretinal proliferation. Ophthalmology 85:584, 1978
43. **Newsome DA, Einaugler RB:** Tonic pupil following retinal detachment surgery. Arch Ophthalmol 86:233, 1971
44. **Norton EWD:** Retinal detachment in aphakia. Trans Am Ophthalmol Soc 61:770, 1963
45. **O'Connor PR:** Absorption of subretinal fluid after non-drainage retinal detachment surgery. Am J Ophthalmol 76:30, 1973
46. **Pemberton JW:** Schiotz applanation disparity following retinal detachment surgery. Arch Ophthalmol 81:534, 1969
47. **Perez RN, Phelps CD, Burton TC:** Angle-closure glaucoma following scleral buckling operations. Trans Am Acad Ophthalmol Otolaryngol 81:247, 1976
48. **Portney GL, Campbell LH, Casebeer JC:** Acquired heterophoria after surgery for retinal detachment. Av J Ophthalmol 73:985, 1972
48a. **Rachal WF, Burton TC:** Changing concepts of failure after retinal detachment surgery. Arch Ophthalmol 97:480, 1979
49. **Robertson DM:** Anterior segment ischemia after segmental episcleral buckling and cryopexy. Am J Ophthalmol 79:871, 1975
49a. **Robertson DM:** Delayed absorption of subretinal fluid after scleral buckling procedures. Am J Ophthalmol 87:57, 1979
50. **Russo CE, Ruiz RS:** Silicone sponge rejection. Arch Ophthalmol 85:647, 1971
51. **Ryan SJ, Goldberg MF:** Anterior segment ischemia following scleral buckling in sickle cell hemoglobinopathy. Am J Ophthalmol 72:35, 1971
52. **Schwartz PL, Pruett RC:** Factors influencing retinal detachment following removal of buckling elements. Arch Ophthalmol 95:804, 1977
53. **Seelenfreund MH, Kraushar, MF, Schepens CL, Freilich DB:** Choroidal detachment associated with primary retinal detachment. Arch Ophthalmol 91:254, 1974
54. **Sewell JJ, Knobloch WH, Eifrig DE:** Extraocular muscle imbalance after treatment for retinal detachment. Am J Ophthalmol 78:321, 1974
55. **Shea M:** Complications common to all surgical procedures. In Schepens CL, Regan CDJ (eds): Controversial Aspects of the Management of Retinal Detachment. Boston, Little, Brown, 1965, p 207
56. **Stratford TP:** Fate of the reattached retina following removal of silicone elements. In Pruett RC, Regan CDJ (eds): Retina Congress. New York, Appleton-Century-Crofts, 1974, p 623
57. **Sudarsky RD, Yanuzzi LA:** Cryomarcation line and pigment migration after retinal cryosurgery. Arch Ophthalmol 83:395, 1970
58. **Tanenbaum HC, Schepens CL, Elzeneiny I, Freeman HM:** Macular pucker following retinal detachment surgery. Arch Ophthalmol 83:286, 1970
59. **Theodossiadis G:** Diplopia after retinal detachment surgery with cryotherapy and episcleral silastic sponges. Klin Monatsbl Augenheilk 166:423, 1975
60. **Townsend R, Benson WE:** Late redetachment of the retina (In press)
61. **Ulrich RA, Burton TC:** Infections following scleral buckling procedures. Arch Ophthalmol 92:213, 1974

10

PROPHYLACTIC
THERAPY*

Autopsy and clinical studies have shown that 5 to 13 per cent[4, 5, 18, 20, 33, 38] of the population have at least one retinal break.† For every person with a retinal detachment, there are 70 with full-thickness breaks. In this chapter, each type of retinal break will be considered from the point of view of prophylactic therapy (Table 10-1).

SYMPTOMATIC‡ TEARS IN PATIENTS WITH NO HISTORY OF RETINAL DISEASE

FLAP (HORSESHOE) TEARS

There is no doubt that flap tears associated with symptoms are dangerous. From 25 to 90 per cent have been found to cause retinal detachment.[11, 13, 30] Prophylactic treatment of symptomatic flap tears reduces the incidence of retinal detachment 0 to 19 per cent.[10, 12, 27, 29, 37, 40, 43] Such treatment therefore seems justified.

OPERCULATED TEARS

Fresh§ operculated tears are less likely to cause detachment than are fresh flap tears because the traction on the retina is released when the operculum is pulled free. Two small studies[11, 13] have shown that one out of six patients with untreated fresh operculated tears will develop a retinal detachment. In evaluating operculated tears for therapy, it is important to examine the vitreous cavity carefully with the Goldmann three-mirror lens. If the vitreous is adherent to the edge of the round hole, the hole should be considered the equivalent of a flap tear and should be treated. Fresh operculated tears should also be treated if they are large, superiorly located, or are associated with significant vitreous hemorrhage.

*Portions of this chapter have been borrowed from Benson, W. E.: Prophylactic treatment of retinal breaks. Surv. Ophthalmol., 22:41, 1977, with the permission of the publisher.

†A "break" is any full-thickness retinal defect. A "tear" is a break caused by vitreous traction. A "hole" is a round break.

‡A symptomatic tear is a tear caused by posterior vitreous detachment in the eye of a patient complaining of light flashes (photopsias) and/or floaters (entopsias). An atrophic round hole in lattice degeneration in a patient with floaters should not be considered to be symptomatic, since it is unrelated to the posterior vitreous detachment.

§A fresh tear is either a symptomatic tear or a tear found in a location where no tear was seen on prior ophthalmic examination.

TABLE 10-1. INDICATIONS FOR PROPHYLACTIC THERAPY

	Fellow eye	Aphakic	Symptomatic	Asymptomatic
Flap tear	Treat	Occasionally Treat	Treat	—
Operculated tear	Treat	Occasionally Treat	Occasionally Treat	—
Round hole	Treat	—	—	—
Lattice degen-eration with or without holes	Treat	—	—	—
Outer wall holes (retinoschisis)	Treat	—	—	Occasionally Treat

ASYMPTOMATIC BREAKS IN PATIENTS WITH NO HISTORY OF RETINAL DISEASE

FLAP TEARS

Eyes with asymptomatic flap tears have a very low incidence of subsequent retinal detachment. Such tears can be followed without treatment.[8, 23, 30]

ROUND HOLES, WITH OR WITHOUT OPERCULUM

These holes have been found to be harmless in several series.[8, 23, 30] There is no evidence that such tears should be treated.

LATTICE DEGENERATION WITHOUT HOLES

Lattice degeneration is a known precursor of retinal detachment, as vitreous traction on its posterior edge may cause a flap tear (see chapter 3, Predisposing Conditions). It is found in approximately 41 per cent of patients who undergo retinal surgery.[1] However, since it is known to be present in nearly 6 per cent of the population,[6, 20] it is apparent that only a small number of individuals with lattice degeneration develop retinal detachment. No treatment is indicated for lattice degeneration without holes.

LATTICE DEGENERATION WITH HOLES

Lattice degeneration with holes is more likely to lead to retinal detachment than is lattice degeneration without holes because fluid may gain access to the subretinal space. Nevertheless, the risk is not great. Of the 66 patients with this entity followed by Byer,[7] none developed a retinal detachment. Therefore, prophylactic therapy of lattice degeneration with holes is not indicated, though the patients should be reexamined at 6-month intervals.

BREAKS IN APHAKIC EYES

Since 2 to 5 per cent of all aphakic eyes develop retinal detachment,[39] they should be carefully examined for retinal breaks and early detachment. Observation is particularly important during the first year following cataract surgery, when 50 per cent of the detachments occur.[1] Several studies have shown that asymptomatic tears and round holes in aphakic eyes can be safely followed without treatment.[19, 24, 30] However, if they are large or posteriorly located, they may warrant treatment.

BREAKS IN FELLOW EYES

PHAKIC FELLOW EYES

The bilateral incidence of retinal detachment is 10 per cent.[14, 16, 21, 26, 41, 44] Davis et al.[14] have compiled the best study on the natural history of the second or "fellow" eyes of patients who have had a retinal detachment in one eye. In their series, 7 of 42 fellow eyes with flap tears, and 0 of 26 with operculated tears developed retinal detachment. They also found that 9 of 38 fellow eyes with lattice degeneration, 11 of 68 with focal pigmented spots, and 4 of 51 with vitreoretinal tags with traction had subsequent retinal detachment in the second eye. Hyams followed 32 fellow eyes which developed fresh tears while under observation.[23] Ten of these had retinal detachment very soon after the advent of the fresh tear. In another study,[26] 19 per cent of 966 fellow eyes had retinal breaks. Twenty per cent of these had subsequent retinal detachment. Clearly, then, patients who have had a retinal detachment in one eye are at high risk of detachment in the second eye. Prophylactic therapy has proven beneficial in the treatment of vitreoretinal abnormalities in these fellow eyes.[12, 27, 34] In Israel,[26, 41] following the introduction of prophylactic therapy, the incidence of retinal detachment in fellow eyes decreased from 11 to 3 per cent.

APHAKIC FELLOW EYES

The incidence of retinal detachment in aphakic fellow eyes is two to three times that of phakic fellow eyes (21 to 36 per cent[2, 9, 14] as compared to 10 per cent). In this very high risk group, prophylactic treatment of all retinal breaks, lattice degeneration, and vitreoretinal tags is beneficial.[2]

FELLOW EYES OF PATIENTS WITH GIANT TEAR

In a study at Moorfields Eye Hospital, 42 per cent of patients with a giant tear (defined as a tear which is 90° or larger) in one eye had a subsequent retinal detachment in the other eye.[25] Since retinal detachments with giant tears are very difficult to repair, prevention of detachment in the second eye is very important. At Moorfields, the peripheral retina of the fellow eye is treated with circumferential cryotherapy, even if it has no clinically apparent vitreoretinal abnormalities. Such treatment seems justified.

BREAKS IN MYOPIC EYES

Because highly myopic eyes are at high risk of retinal detachment, some surgeons treat all breaks found, even asymptomatic round holes (see chapter 3,

Predisposing Conditions). However, two separate studies from Israel have shown that asymptomatic breaks are unlikely to cause a subsequent detachment.[24, 30] It has been estimated that there are 35 myopic eyes with breaks for every myopic eye which develops a retinal detachment.[31] Asymptomatic retinal breaks found in myopic eyes need not be treated.

BREAKS IN SENILE RETINOSCHISIS

On routine autopsy examination of eyes with no history of ocular disease, nearly 1 per cent had senile retinoschisis with outer wall holes.[17] Hirose and colleagues[22] followed a large number of patients with senile retinoschisis in order to determine the natural history of the condition. Retinal detachment did not develop in any of the 25 eyes with outer wall holes, nor in any of the six eyes with both inner and outer wall holes. They also observed an additional 245 cases of retinoschisis without holes. Nine developed outer wall holes during the period of observation; retinal detachment occurred subsequently in three of them. Because of the low incidence of retinal detachment and because retinal detachments caused by retinoschisis progress slowly, it is not necessary to treat all outer wall holes. They should, however, be treated if they are large, multiple, or posteriorly located[22] (Fig. 10-1) or if they are found in the fellow eye of a patient who has had a retinoschisis detachment in the other eye. Fresh breaks should be watched carefully.

SUBCLINICAL RETINAL DETACHMENT

A retinal detachment is called subclinical if subretinal fluid extends at least 1 disc diameter from the retinal break, but no more than 2 disc diameters posterior to the equator (Fig. 10-2A).[13] Thirty per cent of such detachments will progress,[13] so treatment is indicated. A scleral buckling procedure is generally necessary, but if there is little or no vitreous traction, cryotherapy or photocoagulation[34] combined with bed rest may induce settling of the retina and sealing of the break. Treatment should be applied adjacent to the break, but also to a 3 to 4-mm. band of attached retina surrounding the subclinical detachment (Fig. 10-2B). In this way, the detachment may be successfully walled off even if the retina does not settle. It is of critical importance that such treatment extend to the ora serrata to prevent anterior leakage of subretinal fluid. This technique for containing a subclinical detachment may also be tried in the treatment of other types of detachment for patients who refuse or cannot undergo a scleral buckling procedure.

RETINAL BREAKS WITH BRIDGING VESSELS

Generally, when vitreous traction tears the retina, it also tears the retinal vessels crossing the break. In some cases, however, an untorn vessel may cross over, or "bridge," the break. The continued vitreous traction on this vessel can cause recurrent vitreous hemorrhage.[36] It can also pull on the posterior edge of the retinal break (Fig. 10-3). This additional traction may prevent successful treatment of a flap tear by photocoagulation or cryotherapy alone. A patient

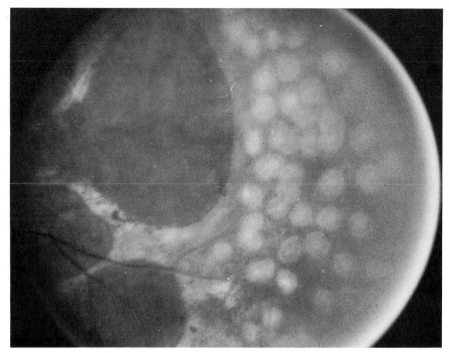

FIG. 10-1. Argon laser prophylactic treatment of posteriorly located, large, outer wall holes in senile retinoschisis. The patient's fellow eye had had a retinoschisis–retinal detachment.

FIG. 10-2. (*A*) Subclinical retinal detachment. (*B*) Walling-off technique used in selected cases (see text). The treatment (*dark band*) must extend 3 to 4 mm. into attached retina and to the ora serrata.

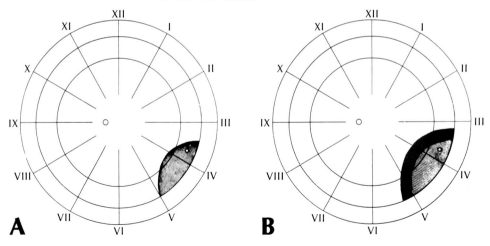

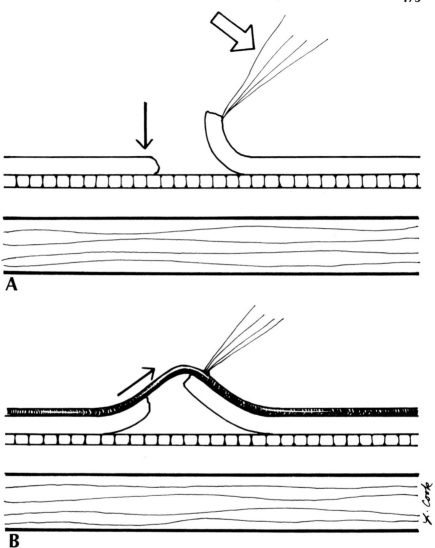

FIG. 10-3. (*A*) Bridging vessels. A flap tear with no bridging vessel. Vitreous traction (*open arrow*) on the flap is not transmitted to the posterior margin of the tear (*arrow*). (*B*) When a vessel bridges a flap tear, vitreous traction is transmitted to the posterior margin. Cryotherapy may not suffice to close the break.

who has been treated with either of these modalities should be examined at intervals of 2 to 3 days until a firm adhesion develops.

MACULAR PUCKER

Macular pucker occurs in 1 to 3 per cent of eyes which have been treated with prophylactic photocoagulation,[28, 40, 42] and in 0 to 1 per cent of eyes treated with cryotherapy.[10, 27, 37] Since pucker can spontaneously occur,[37] especially in eyes with retinal tears, the causative role of the therapy is hard to determine. It seems likely, however, that the therapy can cause pucker in some cases, especially when extensive treatment has been given, as in cases with large areas of lattice degeneration.

TECHNIQUE

Both cryotherapy and photocoagulation (argon laser or xenon arc) are accepted modalities used in the prophylactic treatment of retinal breaks. No matter which is chosen, the cardinal rule of treatment is to adequately surround the break. The most common cause of subsequent retinal detachment is inadequate treatment anterior to flap tears.[3, 37] Continued vitreous traction can extend the flap anteriorly, allowing leakage of subretinal fluid and giving rise to a detachment. Because it is easier to treat anteriorly with cryotherapy, and because cryotherapy is less likely to be followed by macular pucker, it is often preferred to photocoagulation. However, treatment of posterior breaks is easier with photocoagulation.

CRYOTHERAPY

The surgeon should make a careful preoperative drawing so that all breaks will be treated. Proparacaine 1 per cent drops are instilled in both eyes: in the treated eye, so that subsequent cocaine drops will not cause severe pain, and in the untreated eye to diminish photophobia. After 10 per cent cocaine drops have been instilled in the eye to be treated, a cotton pledget soaked in cocaine is placed in the quadrant(s) in which the breaks are located. Usually this will provide sufficient analgesia. If not, subconjunctival xylocaine 1 per cent is injected. Retrobulbar anesthesia is rarely necessary. Most patients are treated as outpatients.[35, 45]

If extensive cryotherapy is planned, the inferior areas should be treated first. Cryotherapy-induced chemosis restricts access to inferior portions of the globe before superior portions because the inferior fornix is much shorter. Operculated and round holes are surrounded with a 2-mm. rim of contiguous cryotherapy. The treatment of flap tears is extended to the ora serrata, lest continued vitreous traction extend them through cryotherapy scars, allowing anterior leakage of subretinal fluid (Fig. 10-4).[3, 37] Finally, the entire retina must be carefully examined with scleral depression so that all possible foci for retinal tears (e.g., vitreoretinal tags, pigmented spots, and prominent meridional folds with posterior thinning) can be treated.

In order to treat a posterior break, "cutting" cryotherapy is necessary. A

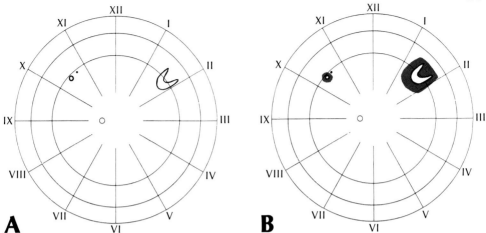

FIG. 10-4. Proper treatment of retinal tears. (*A*) Preoperative drawing. Flap tear at 1:30; operculated tear at 10:30. (*B*) Adequate treatment of the operculated tear, inadequate treatment of the flap tear. Its treatment should extend to the ora serrata. (*C*) Increased vitreous traction has extended the flap tear through the cryotherapy scar. Anterior leakage causes a retinal detachment. (*D*) Properly treated tears. Treatment of the flap tear extends to the ora serrata.

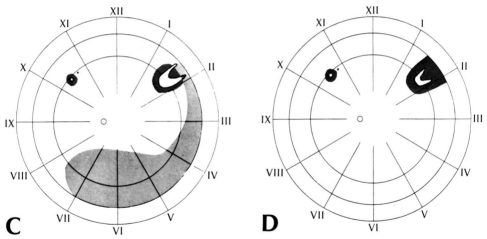

small incision is made in the conjunctiva and Tenon's capsule to allow posterior passage of the cryoprobe.

PHOTOCOAGULATION

Xenon arc or argon laser photocoagulation can also be used to treat retinal breaks. Retrobulbar anesthesia is always required in conjunction with xenon arc and sometimes with argon laser. The break is surrounded by a double or triple row of 4.5° or 500 micron burns (Fig. 10-5). Photocoagulation should not be used to treat flap tears unless the surgeon is skilled enough to extend the treatment to the ora serrata. It is predominantly used in the treatment of posteriorly located breaks, as a less complicated alternative to "cutting" cryotherapy.

It is difficult for the photocoagulation beam to penetrate a cataract or a vitreous hemorrhage. Cryotherapy is preferred for such cases. It is also the preferred treatment for eyes with small pupils because the indirect ophthalmoscope provides better visualization than the viewing systems used in photocoagulation.

THE ROLE OF EDUCATION IN PREVENTING VISUAL LOSS

If a patient is familiar with the symptoms of detachment, he is likely to report promptly after its onset. When he does so, he increases his chances for successful surgical and visual results. Delay may mean the development of macular detachment or early massive periretinal proliferation (MPP). Visual acuity is lost as a result of the former, and retinal reattachment is jeopardized by the latter.

In a large series of phakic retinal detachments, 65 per cent of the maculas had detached.[1] In Davis' study of detachment in fellow phakic eyes,[14] the macula had detached in only 25 per cent. The difference between the two figures seems to be largely caused by the prior experience with retinal detachment of Davis' patients.

Macular detachment is even more common in aphakic eyes. A patient who has unilateral aphakia and is not wearing a contact lens or spectacles may not be aware of visual field loss. Even if the patient is wearing aphakic spectacles, a retinal detachment can advance in the periphery before the visual field provided by the spectacles is reduced. Finally, it is the clinical impression of many retinal surgeons that aphakic retinal detachments spread more quickly than do phakic retinal detachments. In two studies,[1,32] the macula had detached in 83 per cent of eyes with aphakic retinal detachment (ARD). A study of ARD in fellow eyes[2] found the macula to be detached in only 40 per cent. Thus, in both phakic and aphakic retinal detachments, a foreknowledge of the symptoms of detachment results in a lower rate of macular involvement.

Two studies which compare detachments in first eyes with those in fellow eyes prove that this foreknowledge contributes to concomitantly better visual results as well as to a higher rate of reattachment. Davis[14] reattached 91 per cent of patients presenting with retinal detachment in the first eye. On the

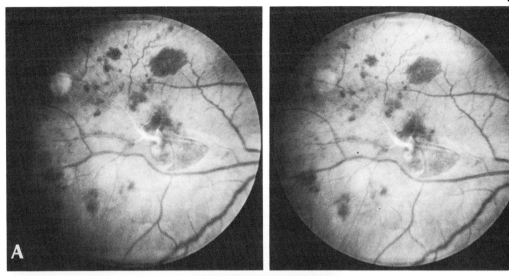

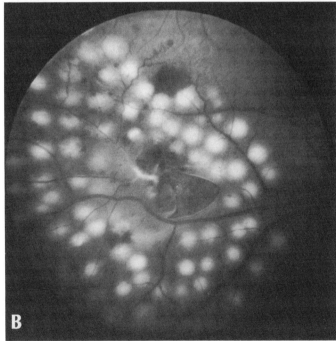

FIG. 10-5. (*A*) Posteriorly located flap tear before treatment (Stereo). (*B*) Same flap tear after photocoagulation. More treatment has been given anteriorly than posteriorly so that the tear will still be contained if traction extends it.

other hand, he successfully reattached 98 per cent of fellow eyes with phakic retinal detachments, and 90 per cent retained a visual acuity of better than 20/50.

Benson and colleagues[2] reported reattachment of 83 per cent of their patients with ARDs in the first eye, with 45 per cent retaining a visual acuity of 20/50 or better. In their series of patients with ARDs in fellow eyes, 96 per cent were successfully reattached, and 72 per cent retained a postoperative acuity of 20/50 or better. Clearly, the patients who had had previous experience with retinal detachment had a much lower incidence of both MPP and macular detachment.

These statistics are very encouraging, for they tell us that the education of patients can affect the outcome of their retinal surgery, both in terms of successful reattachment and visual acuity. All patients at risk of developing retinal detachment—high myopes, aphakes, and patients with lattice degeneration—should be taught the symptoms of detachment and urged to report promptly if any are perceived. They, as well as patients who have already had a detachment, should be trained to check their own peripheral fields at regular intervals.

REFERENCES

1. **Ashrafzadeh MT, Schepens CL, Elzeneiny IH, Moura R, Morse PH, Kraushar MD:** Aphakic and phakic retinal detachment. Arch Ophthalmol 89:476, 1973
2. **Benson WE, Grand MG, Okun E:** Aphakic retinal detachment. Arch Ophthalmol 93:245, 1975
3. **Benson WE, Nantawan P, Morse PH:** Late complications following cryotherapy of lattice degeneration. Am J Ophthalmol 84:514, 1977
4. **Byer NE:** A clinical study of lattice degeneration of the retina. Trans Am Acad Ophthalmol Otolaryngol 69:1064, 1965
5. **Byer NE:** Clinical study of retinal breaks. Trans Am Acad Ophthalmol Otolaryngol 71:461, 1967
6. **Byer NE:** The natural history of the retinopathies of retinal detachment and preventive treatment. In Michaelson IC, Berman ER (eds): Causes and Prevention of Blindness. New York, Academic Press, 1972, pp 397–400
7. **Byer NE:** Changes in and prognosis of lattice degeneration of the retina. Trans Am Acad Ophthalmol Otolaryngol 78:114, 1974
8. **Byer NE:** Prognosis of asymptomatic retinal breaks. Arch Ophthalmol 92:208, 1974
9. **Campbell CJ, Rittler MC:** Cataract extraction in the retinal detachment-prone patient. Am J Ophthalmol 73:17, 1972
10. **Chignell AH, Schilling J:** Prophylaxis of retinal detachment. Br J Ophthalmol 57:291, 1973
11. **Colyear BH, Pischel DK:** Clinical tears in the retina without detachment. Am J Ophthalmol 41:773, 1956
12. **Colyear BH, Pischel DK:** Preventive treatment of retinal detachment by means of light coagulation. Trans Pac Coast Otoophthalmol Soc 41:193, 1960
13. **Davis MD:** The natural history of retinal breaks. Arch Ophthalmol 92:183, 1974
14. **Davis MD, Segal PP, MacCormack A:** The natural course followed by the fellow eye in patients with rhegmatogenous retinal detachment. In Pruett RC, Regan CDJ (eds): Retina Congress. New York, Appleton-Century-Crofts, 1972, pp 643–660
15. **Delaney WV:** Retinal tear extension through the cryosurgical scar. Br J Ophthalmol 55:205, 1971
16. **Dollfus M:** Le traitement préventif du décollement de la rétine. XVIII Concilium Ophthalmologicum, Vol 1. Brussels, Imprimerie Médicale et Scientifique, 1958, pp 988–989

17. **Foos RY:** Senile retinoschisis. Trans Am Acad Ophthalmol Otolaryngol 74:33, 1970
18. **Foos RY:** Posterior vitreous detachment. Trans Am Acad Ophthalmol Otolaryngol 76:480, 1972
19. **Friedman Z, Neumann E, Hyams S:** Vitreous and peripheral retina in aphakia. Br J Ophthalmol 57:52, 1973
20. **Halpern J:** Routine screening of the retinal periphery. Am J Ophthalmol 62:99, 1966
21. **Haut J, Massin M:** Fréquence des décollements de rétine dans la population française. Pourcentage des décollements bilatéraux. Arch Ophthalmol 35:533, 1975
22. **Hirose T, Marcil G, Schepens CL, Freeman HM:** Acquired retinoschisis, observations and treatment. In Pruett RC, Regan CDJ (eds): Retina Congress. New York, Appleton-Century-Crofts, 1972, pp 489–504
23. **Hyams SW, Meir E, Ivry M et al:** Chorioretinal lesions predisposing to retinal detachment. Am J Ophthalmol 78:429, 1974
24. **Hyams SW, Neumann E, Friedman Z:** Myopia-aphakia. II. Vitreous and peripheral retina. Br J Ophthalmol 59:483, 1975
25. **Kanski JJ:** Giant retinal tears. Am J Ophthalmol 79:846, 1975
26. **Merin S, Feiler V, Hyams S et al:** The fate of the fellow eye in retinal detachment. Am J Ophthalmol 71:477, 1971
27. **Morse PH, Scheie HG:** Prophylactic cryoretinopexy of retinal breaks. Arch Ophthalmol 92:204, 1974
28. **Mortimer CB:** The prevention of retinal detachment. Can J Ophthalmol 1:206, 1966
29. **Nadel AJ, Gieser RG:** The treatment of acute horseshoe tears by transconjunctival cryopexy. Ann Ophthalmol 7:1568, 1975
30. **Neumann E, Hyams S:** Conservative management of retinal breaks. A follow-up study of subsequent retinal detachment. Br J Ophthalmol 56:482, 1972
31. **Neumann E, Hyams S, Barkai S et al:** Natural history of retinal holes with specific reference to the development of retinal detachment and the time factor involved. In Michaelson IC, Berman ER (eds): Causes and Prevention of Blindness. New York, Academic Press, 1972, pp. 404–408
32. **Norton EWD:** Retinal detachment in aphakia. Am J Ophthalmol 58:111, 1974
33. **Okun E:** Gross and microscopic pathology of autopsy eyes. Part III. Retinal breaks without detachment. Am J Ophthalmol 51:369, 1961
34. **Okun E, Cibis PA:** Photocoagulation in "limited" retinal detachment and breaks without detachment. In McPherson A (ed): New and Controversial Aspects of Retinal Detachment. New York, Harper & Row, 1968, pp 164–171
35. **Ramsay RC, Eifrig DE:** Outpatient treatment of retinal breaks. Am J Ophthalmol 76:782, 1973
36. **Robertson DM, Curtin VT, Norton EWD:** Avulsed retinal vessels with retinal breaks. Arch Ophthalmol 85:669, 1971
37. **Robertson DM, Norton EWD:** Long-term follow-up of treated retinal breaks. Am J Ophthalmol 75:395, 1973
38. **Rutnin V, Schepens CL:** Fundus appearance in normal eyes. III. Peripheral degenerations. Am J Ophthalmol 64:1040, 1967
39. **Scheie HG, Morse PH, Aminlari A:** Incidence of retinal detachment following cataract extraction. Arch Ophthalmol 89:293, 1973
40. **Sollner F:** Uber die prophylaktische Behandlung der Ablatio retinae durch Lichtcoagulation. Ber Dtsch Ophthalmol Ges 66:327, 1964
41. **Stein R, Feller-Ofry V, Romano A:** The effect of treatment in the prevention of retinal detachment. In Michaelson IC, Berman ER (eds): Causes and Prevention of Blindness. New York, Academic Press, 1972, pp 409–410
42. **Straatsma BR, Allen RA, Christenson RE:** The prophylaxis of retinal detachment. Trans Pac Coast Otoophthal Soc 46:211, 1965
43. **Tasman W, Jaegers KR:** A retrospective study of xenon photocoagulation and cryotherapy in the treatment of retinal breaks. In Pruett RC, Regan CDJ (eds): Retina Congress. New York, Appleton-Century-Crofts, 1972, pp 557–564
44. **Tornquist R:** Bilateral retinal detachment. Acta Ophthalmol (Kbh) 41:126, 1963
45. **Yanoff M:** Prophylactic therapy of retinal breaks. Ann Ophthalmol 9:283, 1977

APPENDIX

This appendix is intended to serve as a guide to the management of various types of retinal detachment and as a review of some of the principles of treatment.

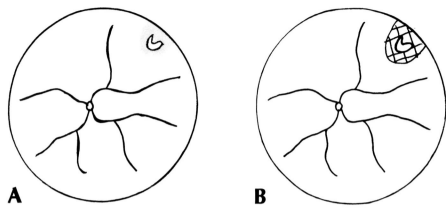

FIG. A-1. *Case 1.* (*A*) Flap tear with small rim of subretinal fluid. (*B*) Cryotherapy without scleral buckling sufficed to seal the break. If the surgeon elects to treat such a case with cryotherapy alone, he must examine the patient at close intervals until the retina is flat. In some cases, the detachment may spread before the cryotherapy scar is firm.

FIG. A-2. *Case 2.* (*A*) Flap tear with more extensive retinal detachment than was present in Case 1. (Or, Case 1, if the cryotherapy alone failed to seal the break.) (*B*) Treatment with a radial sponge and cryotherapy. Radial sponges cause less "fishmouthing" of flap tears than do circumferential sponges.

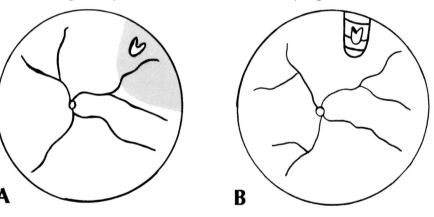

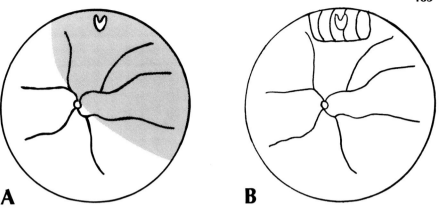

FIG. A-3. *Case 3.* (*A*) Retinal detachment caused by a flap tear under the superior rectus muscle. (*B*) To avoid placing excessive sponge material under the superior rectus muscle, a circumferential, rather than a radial, sponge is used.

FIG. A-4. *Case 4.* (*A*) Retinal detachment caused by an inferotemporal dialysis. (*B*) Treatment with a circumferential sponge explant and cryotherapy.

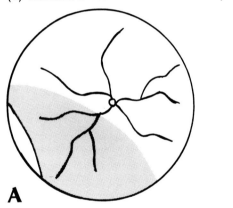
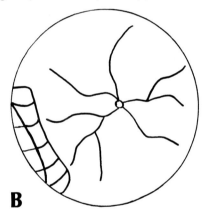

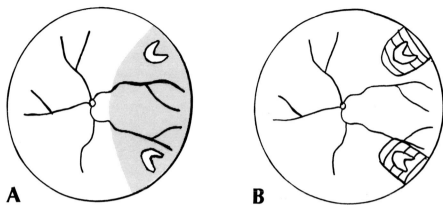

FIG. A-5. *Case 5.* (*A*) Retinal detachment caused by two flap tears. (*B*) Treatment with two radial sponges and cryotherapy.

FIG. A-6. *Case 6.* (A) Retinal detachment caused by two flap tears, which are too close together to be treated by separate radial sponges. (*B*) Treatment with a circumferential explant and cryotherapy.

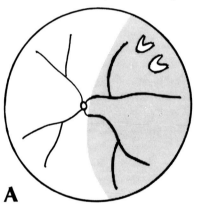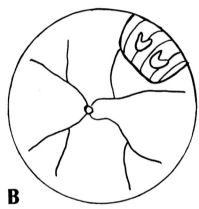

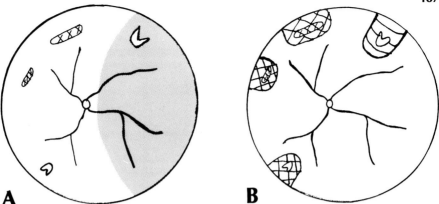

A   **B**

FIG. A-7. *Case 7.* (A) Retinal detachment caused by a superotemporal flap tear. Two patches of lattice degeneration and a flap tear are present in attached retina. (B) The flap tear causing the detachment is treated with a radial sponge and cryotherapy. The other abnormalities are treated with cryotherapy to prevent late redetachment.

FIG. A-8. *Case 8.* (A) Total retinal detachment caused by a flap tear and three round holes. (B) The flap tear is closed by a radial sponge; the round holes by an encircling band. Alternatively, the round holes could have been closed by a segmental circumferential sponge.

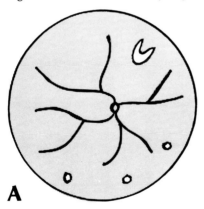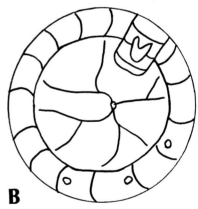

A   **B**

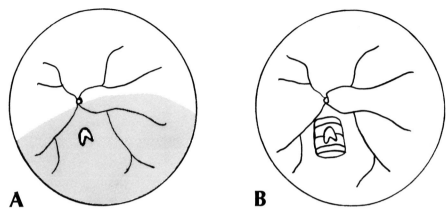

FIG. A-9. *Case 9.* (*A*) Retinal detachment caused by a posterior flap tear. (*B*) Treatment with a radial sponge and cryotherapy. It is easier to place posterior sutures for radial sponges than for circumferential ones.

FIG. A-10. *Case 1.* (*A*) Aphakic retinal detachment caused by four small flap tears at the posterior vitreous base. (*B*) Treatment with an encircling silicone band and cryotherapy. An encircling element is indicated in most aphakic retinal detachments to close undetected breaks and to prevent redetachment. The incidence of massive periretinal proliferation is higher in aphakic than in phakic eyes.

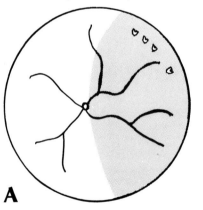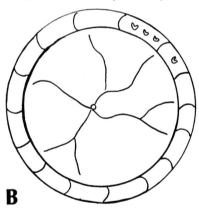

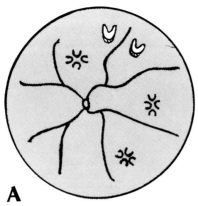
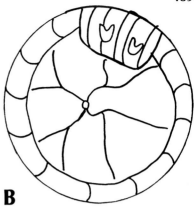

A **B**

FIG. A-11. *Case 11.* (A) Retinal detachment caused by two flap tears. Early massive periretinal proliferation is indicated by the posteriorly rolled edges of the tears and by the three fixed folds. (B) The tears are closed by a circumferential explant and cryotherapy. An encircling band helps to counter vitreous traction.

FIG. A-12. *Case 12.* (A) Failure to reattach the retina. The temporal edge of the flap tear is not supported by the buckle. (B) The retina is reattached by a correctly placed sponge.

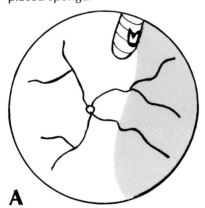
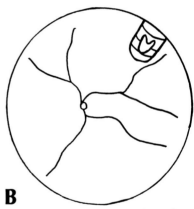

A **B**

FIG. A-13. *Case 13.* (A) Failure to reattach the retina. The sponge explant does not support the anterior horns of the flap tear. (B) The retina is reattached by a slightly larger sponge.

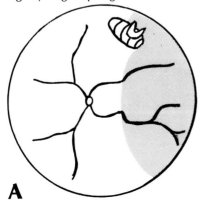
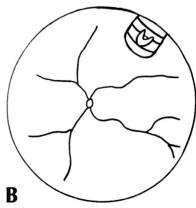

A **B**

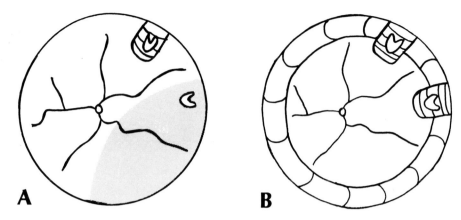

FIG. A-14. *Case 14.* (*A*) Redetachment of the retina caused by a new flap tear. (*B*) The new tear is closed by a radial sponge. Because the new tear indicates increased vitreous traction, an encircling band is added.

FIG. A-15. *Case 15.* (*A*) Redetachment of the retina caused by a new flap tear posterior to the original buckle. (*B*) The retina is reattached by a radial sponge and cryotherapy.

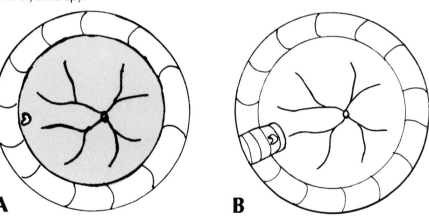

INDEX

Numerals in *italics* indicate a figure; "t" following a page number indicates a table.